MILADY Teaching Hair Coloring:
A Step-by-Step Guide to Building Props

MILADY Teaching Hair Coloring: A Step-by-Step Guide to Building Props

Andre Nizetich

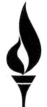

Milady Publishing Company
(A Division of Delmar Publishers Inc.)
3 Columbia Circle, Box 12519
Albany, New York 12212-2519

NOTICE TO THE READER

Publisher does not warrant or guarantee any of the products described herein or perform any independent analysis in connection with any of the product information contained herein. Publisher does not assume, and expressly disclaims, any obligation to obtain and include information other than that provided to it by the manufacturer.

The reader is expressly warned to consider and adopt all safety precautions that might be indicated by the activities described herein and to avoid all potential hazards. By following the instructions contained herein, the reader willingly assumes all risks in connection with such instructions.

The publisher makes no representations or warranties of any kind, including but not limited to, the warranties of fitness for particular purpose or merchantability, nor are any such representations implied with respect to the material set forth herein, and the publisher takes no responsibility with respect to such material. The publisher shall not be liable for any special, consequential or exemplary damages resulting, in whole or in part, from the readers' use of, or reliance upon, this material.

Credits:
  Senior Administrative Editor: Catherine Frangie
  Developmental Editor: Joseph Miranda
  Freelance Project Editor: Pamela Fuller
  Production Manager: John Mickelbank
  Cover Design and Illustration: Gamut Production

COPYRIGHT © 1993
by Milady Publishing Co.
a division of Delmar Publishers Inc.

All rights reserved. No part of this work covered by the copyright hereon may be reproduced or used in any form or by any means — graphic, electronic, or mechanical, including photocopying, recording, taping, or information storage and retrieval systems — without written permission of the publisher.

Printed in the United States of America

1 2 3 4 5 6 7 8 9 10 XXX 99 98 97 96 95 94 93

Library of Congress Cataloging-in-Publication Data:

Nizetich, Andre.
  Teaching hair coloring: a step-by-step guide to building props.
    p. cm.
  ISBN: 1-56253-072-0 (textbook)
  1. Hair — Dyeing and bleaching. I. Title.
TT973.N39 1993
646.7'242–dc20

92-35110
CIP

Contents

Preface vii

PART 1 *The Chemistry of Hair Coloring* 1

- CHAPTER 1   Level System Tint Bottle Prop 3
- CHAPTER 2   Lift/Deposit Chart 6
- CHAPTER 3   The Intensity of Color in the Level System ... 9
- CHAPTER 4   Color Separation 12
- CHAPTER 5   How Peroxide Works 16
- CHAPTER 6   How Volumes of Peroxide React 21
- CHAPTER 7   Using Cloth to Measure Hair Color 24

PART 2 *Physiological Aspects of Hair Color* 27

- CHAPTER 8   Using Your Thumbnail to Describe How Hair Color Works 28
- CHAPTER 9   Cuticle Construction 30
- CHAPTER 10   The Giant Hair Strand 33
- CHAPTER 11   Chocolate Chip Cookies 39
- CHAPTER 12   The King Crab Leg 41
- CHAPTER 13   The Slinky Hair Strand 43
- CHAPTER 14   The Giant Melanin 49
- CHAPTER 15   Dissolving Melanin in the Cortex 53
- CHAPTER 16   Bleaching Dissolving Melanin 58
- CHAPTER 17   Wrap-Around Cuticle 62
- CHAPTER 18   The Decolorization Process 65
- CHAPTER 19   Fast vs. Slow Bleaching 69

| CHAPTER 20 | How Porosity Affects Hair Color | 74 |
| CHAPTER 21 | How the Hair Reflects Color | 81 |

PART 3 The Psychology of Hair Color ... 87

CHAPTER 22	Hair-Color Category Charts	88
CHAPTER 23	Natural Hair-Color Badges	99
CHAPTER 24	The Consultation Book	101

PART 4 Creative Aspects of Hair Coloring ... 105

CHAPTER 25	Making Swatches for Experiments	106
CHAPTER 26	Hair-Color Chart	110
CHAPTER 27	Shuffling Cards	122
CHAPTER 28	Dimensional Hair-Coloring Prop	125
CHAPTER 29	Creating Different Hair Colors with Dimensional Hair Coloring	132
CHAPTER 30	Coloring Gray Hair	136

Hair Coloring Glossary ... 144

Preface

You stand in front of a class of students and explain how hair coloring works. Everything is going just fine. You start by talking about the temporary colors, explaining how the colors coat the hair and how they start to come off the next time that the hair gets shampooed. You pour out some of the colors on a paper towel, and the color that you see matches pretty closely the name of the color. You pour out "Silver Lining" and you see blue, you pour out "Plush Brown" and you see brown, and so on with the temporary colors. It's pretty much the same with the semipermanent colors; whatever name is on the bottle is what you see when you pour it out.

Now comes the tough part, explaining to your students what makes the peroxide/permanent colors work. What's in the bottle? What does it do to the hair? Where is it deposited? Why does it change colors? As you attempt to explain how the permanent colors work, you see a mass of wrinkled foreheads; your students are not quite understanding what you are talking about. Why don't they understand? You are explaining the same way it was explained to you. After all, this is not brain surgery. They should be able to understand it.

It is frustrating to try to teach someone something and not be able to reach them. You use a sequence of words arranged in a variety of ways to attempt to enlighten them, but to no avail.

Some things are just better explained with props. My own frustration with teaching prompted me to write this book on how to build a variety of props to use for teaching hair coloring.

You can only really learn to color hair by doing it. It is like trying to learn to dance without music. Or have someone describe the flavor of an avocado to you and not being able to taste it. The transfer of knowledge is difficult, particularly when it comes to describing what happens with hair color. The more props that you have at your disposal to aid you in transferring that knowledge, the more enjoyable the process will become for both you and your students.

The props that I have included in this book complement my own philosophy of how to teach hair coloring. Some of the props you will embrace, and some you will no doubt disregard because they do not fit into your method of teaching hair coloring. If you use just one of these props and, as a result of its use, you help just one student to better understand hair coloring, both your time and mine will have been well spent.

Andre Nizetich

PART 1

The Chemistry of Hair Coloring

CHAPTER 1
Level System Tint Bottle Prop

Learning hair coloring can be confusing for the cosmetology student. Using props to illustrate the various aspects of hair color can make the subject a little less threatening for the student and easier for the instructor. We start our prop building odyssey with perhaps the most basic and consistent topic — the chemistry of hair color.

The chemistry of hair color is governed by an established set of rules and guidelines that remain consistent regardless of which brand of hair coloring product you are working with. Therefore, the chemistry of hair color is usually one of the easiest topics to convey to students. Although each line of hair color is slightly different, they all work basically the same way. For example, you can say with confidence that if you raise the volume of peroxide you will get additional lifting action, regardless of which brand you are using.

Several props can be easily made that will help reinforce to the cosmetology student a better understanding of the chemistry of hair coloring. It is not important that they know in detail what the active ingredients are in a bottle of hair color. What is important is how a bottle of hair color works, the chemical action that takes place, and what the ingredients in the bottle or tube are capable of performing.

A certain mystery surrounds peroxide/permanent hair colors. Most peroxide colors look nothing like the label indicates when they are poured out on a towel. The mystery is further reinforced because the tint changes when it is mixed with peroxide, then changes further when it is applied to the hair. Therefore the cosmetology instructor should explain exactly what occurs during the oxidation process.

The level system has been adopted by all professional hair color companies as the accepted method of determining the lift/deposit ratio in a bottle or tube of hair color. The best method of illustrating this to your students is to build the following prop.

Assemble the necessary materials for building the prop. Depending on the level system that you intend to use, gather that number of bottles (0-10, 11 bottles; 0-12, 13 bottles; 1-10, 10 bottles). Here we are going to use the level system from 0-10. We are, therefore, going to need 11 bottles. Very few hair color manufacturers package their hair coloring in clear bottles. The bottles pictured here are from TORRID blonde shades manufactured by Clairol.

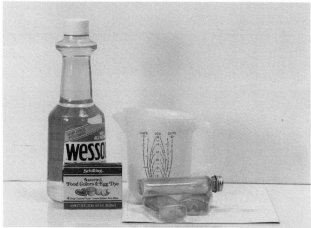

Figure 1.1

You will need some type of oil, plastic numbers (the stick-on type that come on a sheet and can be purchased at the stationery store), 11 empty hair-coloring bottles, and food coloring (food coloring works best — it tends not to separate as do some of the poster paints and water colors — and the colors remain consistent). A small funnel is helpful, as is a large mixing cup with a pour spout. Soak the empty bottles in hot, soapy water, so you can easily peel off the labels and any excess glue.

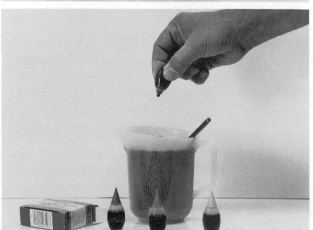

Figure 1.2

Pour 14 ounces of clean water into the mixing cup. Alternately add blue, yellow, and red food coloring to the water until you get a dark, muddy color.

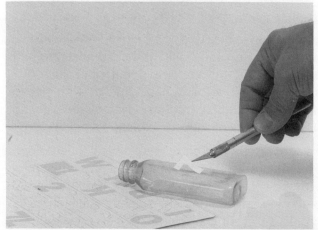

Figure 1.3

Place corresponding numbers on the bottles. An attempt should be made to place the numbers in the same place on the bottles. A cardboard template will assist you in accomplishing this.

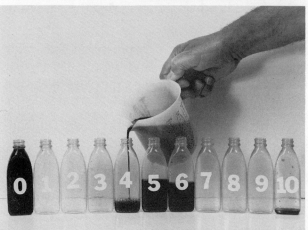

Figure 1.4

Start in the middle range of the levels and fill the bottle half full. Work in each direction, and increase the amount of color as you move toward the smaller numbers and decrease the amount of color as you move toward the larger numbers that were placed in each bottle.

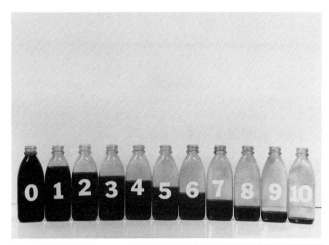

Figure 1.5
Continue pouring small amounts of color from one bottle to the next until you have evenly spaced increments between each bottle.

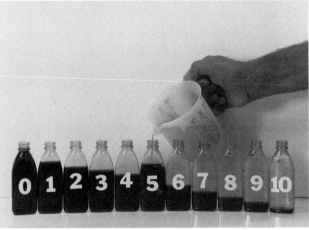

Figure 1.6
Fill each bottle with oil. Fill to the very top so that there is no air remaining in the bottles. Seal top firmly.

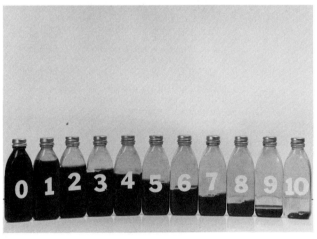

Figure 1.7
You have a valuable tool that can be used to illustrate the lift/deposit ratio in the level system.

Explain to your students that not all level systems are the same; for instance, Wella level 5 and Goldwell level 5 are not the same colors. Each line of hair color is slightly different. It is, therefore, important to emphasize that in the beginning the student should learn one line of hair color well rather than to attempt to learn many lines.

With this prop the student can more clearly see how a bottle of hair color works.

CHAPTER 2

Lift/Deposit Chart

How a hair-coloring product reacts to the hair can be mystifying for the student. This prop helps to demystify the relationship between the lift portion of a bottle/tube of hair color and the deposit portion. By understanding this relationship, the student will come to grips with the limitations of a hair-coloring product.

Many hair-color practitioners have the false impression that it is possible to achieve the maximum amount of lift and at the same time achieve the maximum amount of deposit. Using this prop will give a clear picture of what actually occurs.

LIFT/DEPOSIT CHART

Figure 2.1

Mark an 11 x 14-in. piece of cardboard as indicated. Draw a straight line across the cardboard 1 1/2 in. from the top. Draw two vertical lines on either side of the cardboard 1 in. from each edge. On the two vertical lines starting at the top, measure down 1 in. and make a mark. Starting with that mark, measure down 5/8 in. and make a series of marks 5/8 in. apart. Make all the marks very lightly with a pencil.

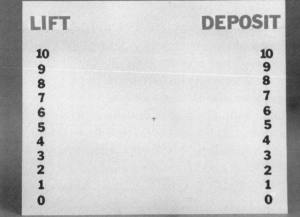

Figure 2.2

With stick-on letters place the words "LIFT" and "DEPOSIT" above the two vertical lines. The words should be the same distance from the edge of the cardboard. Therefore, for the word "DEPOSIT," start with the letter "T," position it, then work towards the center. These stick-on letters can be purchased at a stationery store or any other store that sells school supplies. Place the numbers on the marks on the two verical lines. Use slightly larger, different color letters for the names at the top. Once all the letters and numbers are in place, mark a small cross halfway between the two 6s and the two 5s. This marks the position where the arrow is to be anchored.

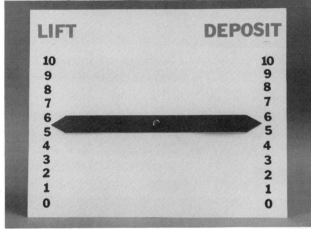

Figure 2.3

Cut a dual arrow out of a small piece of black cardboard. The arrow should be just long enough so that it comes just to the edge of the numbers, and about 3/4 in. wide. Make a mark in the center of the arrow. With a sharp object drill a small hole through the arrow and the cardboard.

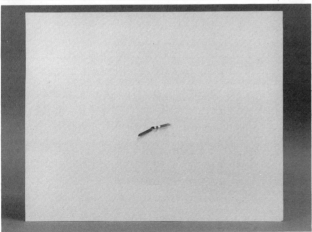

Figure 2.4

Use a paper brad to attach the arrow to the cardboard. Fold the brad over without making it too snug, so that the arrow can move freely.

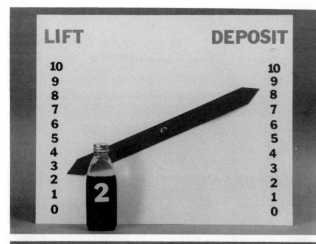

Figure 2.5

This prop may be used in conjunction with the lift/deposit bottles. The bottle is placed in front of the lift/deposit chart so that the student can see how the bottle of color works. For example, suppose you have a bottle of level 2 color. The level numbers are on the lift side of this chart. Point the arrow at the number that corresponds to the number on the bottle. Now by looking over to the deposit side you can see how much deposit you will get with this particular bottle of hair color.

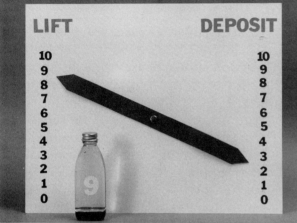

Figure 2.6

Here is an example with a bottle of color that is a level number 9. Level number 9 would be considered a fairly light blonde. Notice that when we put the arrow on number 9 on the lift side, the deposit side registers a low number, indicating a minimum amount of color deposit in this bottle. Therefore it would not be in the best interest of your client to continually comb this small amount of color through the ends of the hair. This could result in the hair becoming damaged. You must remember that the lift portion of a bottle of color acts the same as bleach.

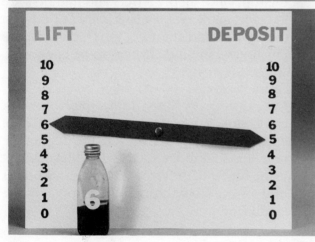

Figure 2.7

Now you show a bottle of color that is a level number 6. You always relate the level number to the lift side of the chart. In this bottle of color there is a fair degree of deposit. A level 6 is dark blonde to light brown in color. When you apply hair color to the hair you must consider the color of hair on which you are applying it. If you are applying a light brown color on medium or darker brown hair the color deposit will not show. You will only get a small amount of lift.

The size of the prop can vary depending on the size of the class. As you enlarge the size of the cardboard you are using, the letters and numbers should enlarge in proportion. Should you enlarge the size of the prop any more than indicated, the cardboard should be at least as thick as matting cardboard. This type of cardboard is available at framing, art supply, and photography stores.

CHAPTER 3

The Intensity of Color in the Level System

This prop is to be used along with the bottles that describe the level system. These bottles are to be used to show the intensity of color at the various levels. The combination of this prop and the bottles describing the level system will give the reader greater insight into how hair-color products work.

10 CHAPTER 3

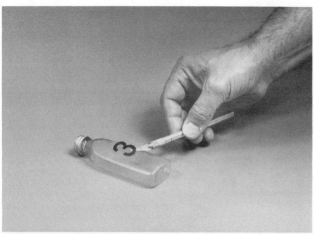

Figure 3.1
Place the numbers 0 through 10 on eleven bottles. This will match exactly the tint bottle prop.

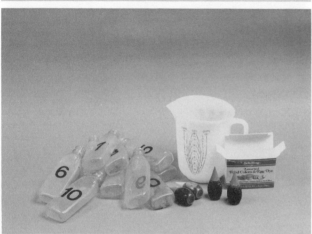

Figure 3.2
Gather the necessary equipment to complete this prop: eleven bottles, food coloring, a 16-ounce measuring cup, and an eye dropper.

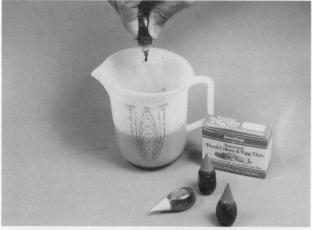

Figure 3.3
Fill the measuring cup with 9 ounces of water. Add blue, yellow, red, and green food coloring to the water, creating a muddy brown color. It will require a substantial amount of food coloring to color the water deeply enough.

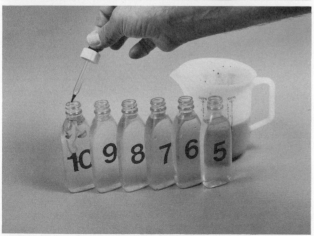

Figure 3.4
Fill bottles 5 through 10 almost to the top with water. Starting with bottle number 10, add a couple of drops to the prepared colored water, to slightly discolor the water.

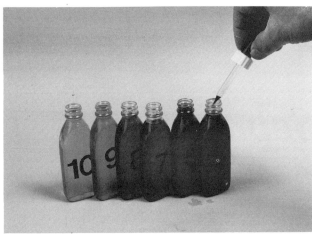

Figure 3.5

Continue to add just slightly more color to each new bottle as you move down the line so it will be slightly darker than the previous bottle.

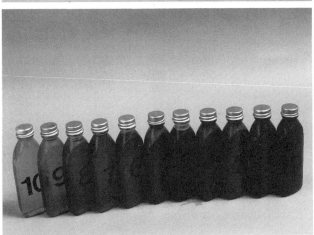

Figure 3.6

Continue this process until level 0 is filled with a dark, solid color. It is difficult to achieve a gradual darkness in the bottles. You will end up spilling out color and refilling the bottles with water to achieve a lighter shade.

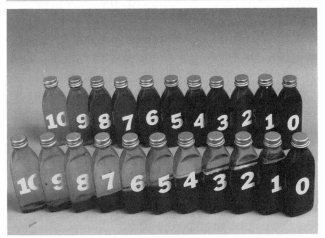

Figure 3.7

Here you see the completed bottles next to the level system tint bottle prop. It became apparent that the use of black numbers were not the most visible means of identifying the bottles, so the numbers were changed to white.

CHAPTER 4
Color Separation

Many of the hair-color classes I have attended start out by talking about the "Laws of Color," how primaries, secondaries, and tertiaries are blended to form all of the colors. The problem is that it is never satisfactorily explained how the Laws of Color relate to hair color. The Laws of Color only work if you can actually see the colors. Our medium is not that simple. We are working with colors that we cannot see. It can be very confusing. The medium that we work on is not like a piece of canvas. The colors that we use change as we mix and apply them. They are never constant. This is why cosmetology instructors should make every effort to help the student understand how the Laws of Color relate to hair color.

Let's start by building a prop that will demonstrate what is in the colors that we work with. The manufacturer's hair color chart is a valuable tool for formulating hair color. I use a color chart to compare one color with another, never to determine what the hair color result will be.

It helps to know what primary colors are used to make a particular shade. This prop is used for that reason. It is easy and not very expensive to make, providing you do it yourself. If you have a professional photographer make it for you it will cost more.

When I teach hair color, I look to other industries that use color to help me with teaching aids. This is where I got the idea for this prop. When I was in the process of writing the book *The Simplified Approach to Haircolor*, the publisher asked if I would check some colors for their accuracy before the pages were printed. Of course, I agreed. When I received the pages they were in the form of, what they call in the printing industry, color separations. When I saw them I thought, "This is great; now I can show my classes how much of each primary color is in each shade of hair color."

I use this prop in conjunction with another prop from the printing industry called "DIAL-A-COLOR." This is a tool that printers use to help them to mix inks and to aid them in determining what percentage of each primary color is in a printed piece.

To make the color separation, select the manufacturer whose hair colors you would like to represent. If a color swatch chart is already available, disregard Figures 4.1 to 4.4.

COLOR SEPARATION **13**

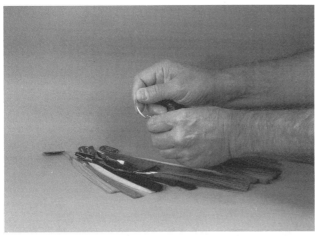

Figure 4.1
Disassemble a manufacturer's sample hair-color ring by pulling off each swatch from the ring that is holding them.

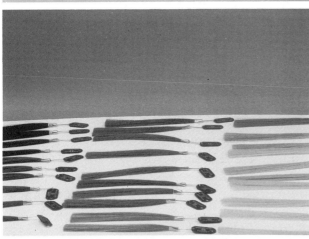

Figure 4.2
Locate a foam core board large enough to accommodate the swatches you would like to mount. The foam core board can be purchased from a picture frame shop or a photo store. Place the swatches in order from lightest to darkest.

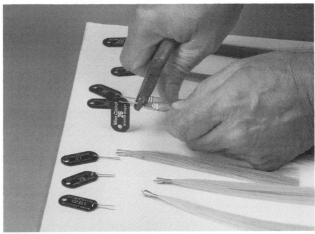

Figure 4.3
Cut the color identification tags from each.

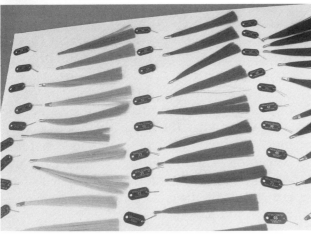

Figure 4.4
Once the tags are removed from the swatches be certain that you do not get the tags and swatches mixed.

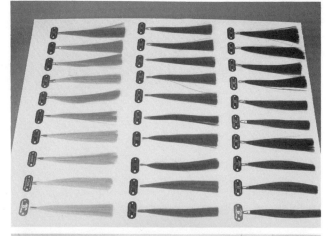

Figure 4.5

Line up the swatches and tags neatly. Photograph the swatches with a quality camera. If you don't have a quality camera, borrow one from a friend. Shoot the swatches in a variety of exposures. Once you get the photographs developed you can determine which exposure gives the most accurate rendering of the colors. Shoot the board using slide film. Once you have determined the slide that gives you the most accurate rendering take the slide to a photo shop or to someone who does color printing and ask for a color separation. You can obtain the separation in whatever size you need for your class. If you are going to use the slide with an overhead projector you can get by with a smaller separation.

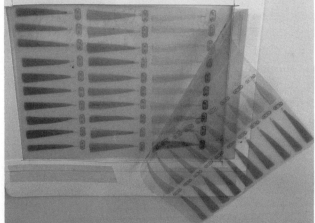

Figure 4.6

Use the color separation to show your class how primary colors are used to make the wide range of hair colors. With the DIAL-A-COLOR you can have the class actually build the colors. You will find, as I have, that your class will understand the Laws of Color and how they relate to hair color after this exercise.

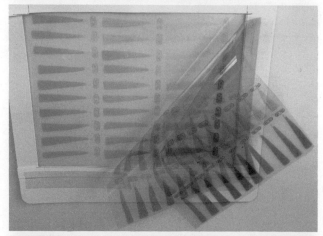

Figure 4.7

With the color separation on the overhead projector, first remove the blue sheet, then remove the red sheet, leaving the yellow. When you perform this exercise using the color separation sheets, your students will quickly learn how the Laws of Color relate to hair coloring.

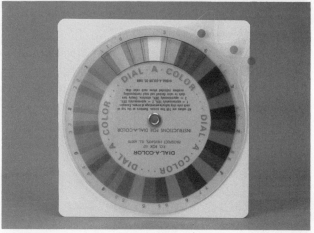

Figure 4.8

The DIAL-A-COLOR is an instrument that is used to determine how much of each primary color is used to make a color. It is used in the printing industry for mixing inks. The printing industry is somewhat like the hair-color industry in that the color ink used is very much affected by the color of paper that it is placed on. The big difference is that the ink does not alter the color of the paper as hair color does the hair.

COLOR SEPARATION 15

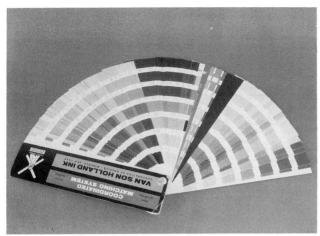

Figure 4.9

Another printing tool that I use to show color variations in hair colors is the Pantone ink chart. It shows a number of colored inks and the formulas that are used to achieve them. Have your students use the DIAL-A-COLOR in conjunction with the Pantone chart to create color variations.

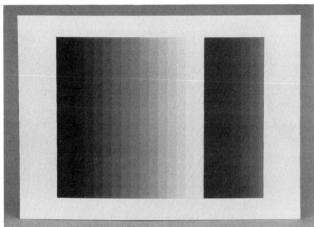

Figure 4.10

This is a level system chart that is used in television production. This is another example of how the level system is used in many industries to show the degrees between black and white or light and dark.

CHAPTER 5

How Peroxide Works

I like to start this session by reading the label on a bottle of peroxide that was purchased at a drugstore for medicinal purposes. First I read the label, then I ask the class if you can use 3 percent peroxide for processing hair color. Then I ask, "What is the difference between percent and volume?" Of course at this point their interest is aroused, and I proceed with the lecture. I have found that very few individuals understand the difference between percent and volume. The following props will help give a clear picture of what peroxide actually is. It is important as colorists that we have a complete understanding of the chemicals we are working with.

The other day I was reading a hair-coloring article on how to achieve a beautiful shaded effect. The article was written by a famous hair colorist from England. All of the formulas in the article used to achieve this particular effect were given with the peroxides stated in percentages. Had I not known the difference between volume and percent the article would have made no sense.

This is a simple enough demonstration to do. No special preparation is necessary. The materials needed to complete the first part of this demonstration are one tall glass, a round piece of Styrofoam, and a product used to produce bubbles, such as liquid soap, detergent, or bubble bath.

HOW PEROXIDE WORKS 17

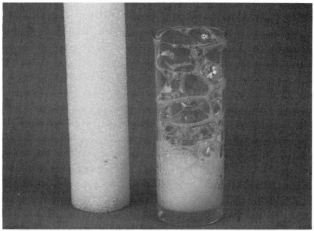

Figure 5.1

Pour into a clean, tall glass (straight-sided glasses are preferred) a small amount of water and a small amount of bubble liquid. Shake the ingredients vigorously until the glass fills with bubbles. At this point explain to the class that what you see is the volume of oxygen. We use bubbles so that we can illustrate to you what one volume looks like. The size of the container is irrelevant; it could be a gallon or it could be a drum; one volume is a container filled with air.

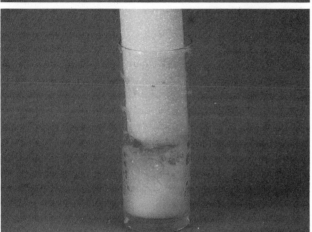

Figure 5.2

Now condense the bubbles to the bottom of the glass by compressing the air with the Styrofoam ram.

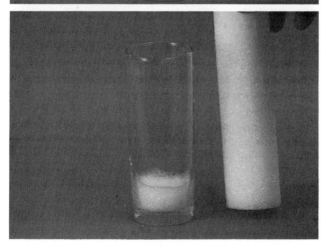

Figure 5.3

Remove the ram from the glass, and show how all of the bubbles have been condensed.

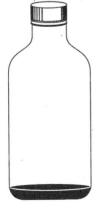

ONE VOLUME

Figure 5.4

After this first step is complete, go to the blackboard, overhead projector, or flip chart, draw a picture of a bottle, and indicate the level the air has been squeezed. This represents one volume.

18 CHAPTER 5

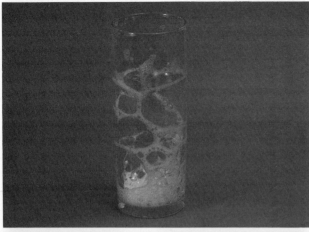

Figure 5.5
Shake the glass again, producing another glass of bubbles.

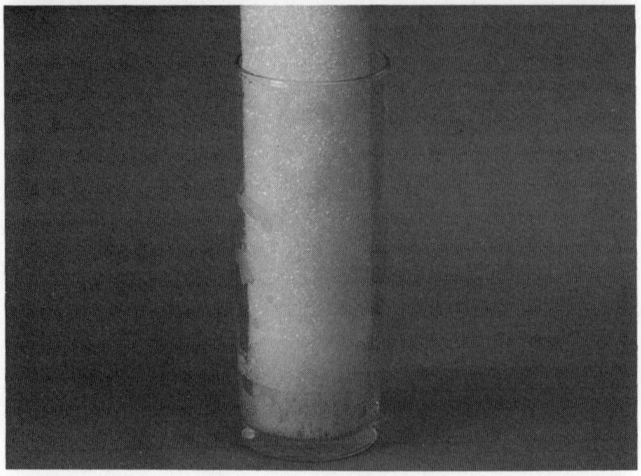

Figure 5.6
Repeat the ramming process again, pushing the Styrofoam ram down to the bottom of the glass.

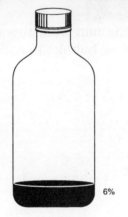

Figure 5.7
Now go to the graph and explain that two volumes of oxygen have been squeezed into the bottom of this glass. If you do this twenty times, you squeeze twenty volumes of air into this glass. What percent peroxide do you have here? You have 6 percent peroxide. That means that all of the oxygen that was squeezed into the bottom of this container takes up 6 percent of the container, thus the term 6 percent peroxide. What volume is a container that indicates 3 percent? It is 10 volume, or half of 6 percent. What percent do you have for every 10 volumes? Continue until you have given the class a good indication of what percent and volume are.

HOW PEROXIDE WORKS

The second part of this experiment also deals with the volume and percent of peroxide. The student should understand the difference between lower volume peroxide and stronger volume peroxide. It is not the oxygen that is condensed into the bottle that renders the peroxide an unstable solution. What makes peroxide an unstable solution is the oxygen that is attempting to escape. The more oxygen that is contained in the container, the greater its capacity to lift color from the hair. This portion of the lecture will give the student a visual picture of the vast difference in the various volumes of peroxide.

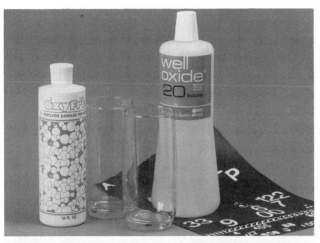

Figure 5.8

The materials that will be needed for this portion of the prop are two tall glasses, stick-on letters, 20 volume peroxide, and a bottle of Oxyfree. Oxyfree releases the oxygen in a more efficient manner than does any other product tested.

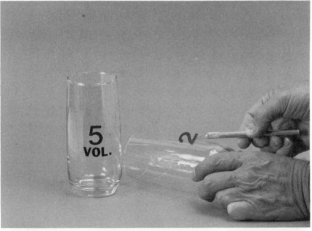

Figure 5.9

Place the number 20, indicating 20 volume peroxide, on one glass. On the other glass place the number 5, to indicate 5 volume peroxide. An attempt should be made to place the numbers in the same position on both of the glasses. If you want to make a more dramatic difference in the visual effect, you may choose to have even a greater spread in the volumes of peroxides.

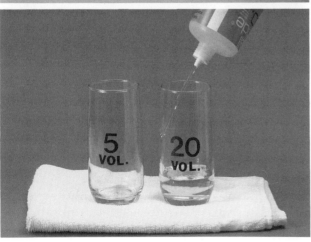

Figure 5.10

Pour some 20 volume peroxide into one glass. Into the other glass pour some 5 volume peroxide (1 oz. of 20 volume peroxide and 3 oz. of water). They both look the same. In the previous experiment we explained the differences in the volumes of peroxide. Now you will more clearly see the differences in the volumes of peroxide.

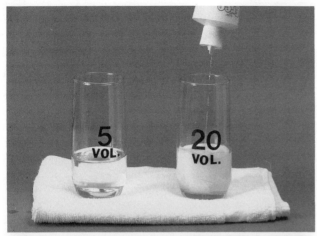

Figure 5.11

Oxyfree is a product that is formulated to get rid of any excess peroxide that is left in the hair after a treatment. When you look at peroxide it looks identical to water. You certainly cannot tell by looking how strong the peroxide is. Pour an equal amount of Oxyfree into each glass. This is going to release all of the oxygen that has been condensed into this liquid.

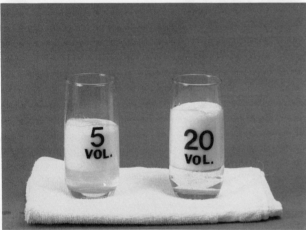

Figure 5.12

You will begin to see all of the oxygen escaping from the liquid. This will give you some idea of the strength in peroxide. Notice the bubbling action that is taking place. Think about each one of these bubbles as being able to carry out of the hair strand one unit of melanin. The more bubbles, the more melanin it can carry away. Now both of these will stop working at the same time. How can that be, you ask? If one is much stronger, won't it react longer? The answer is that it reacts stronger but for the same amount of time. This will continue working until the peroxide has been turned to water.

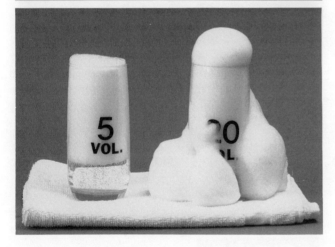

Figure 5.13

Here you see all of the oxygen removed. Notice the difference between the 5 volume and the 20 volume. You can clearly see how much more strength the 20 volume peroxide has. I hope this experiment helps you better understand how peroxide works and the strength that it has. The student will gain much more respect for peroxide when using it with hair coloring.

CHAPTER 6

How Volumes of Peroxide React

It is often confusing to students how peroxide reacts based on the various volumes of peroxides. The strength of peroxide depends largely on the amount of oxygen that is condensed into the liquid. This prop is designed to show how the peroxide dissipates depending on its strength. There is a misconception that the length of time it takes to dissipate 40 volume peroxide is twice as long as it takes to dissipate 20 volume peroxide. The fact is, peroxides of different strengths dissipate at the same time, but with different intensities. This prop will clarify how this works and what it means.

CHAPTER 6

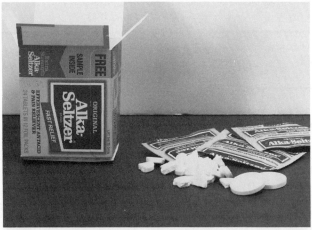

Figure 6.1
Break up several tablets of Alka-Seltzer® into quarters. Fifteen quarters will be required to complete this prop.

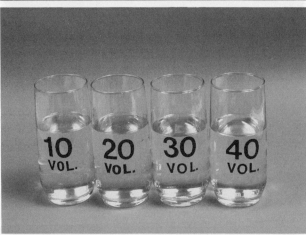

Figure 6.2
As was done with other props using glasses to demonstrate peroxides, place the appropriate numbers on four glasses. Fill the glasses two-thirds full of water.

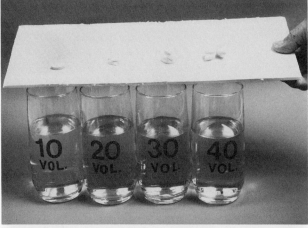

Figure 6.3
Place a piece of cardboard over the glasses. Over the opening of each of the glasses place a quarter of an Alka-Seltzer® for the 10 volume, two quarters for the 20 volume, three quarters for the 30 volume, and four quarters for the 40 volume.

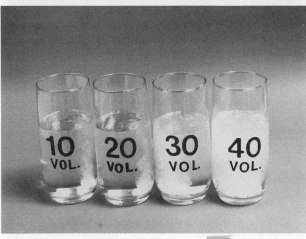

Figure 6.4
Simultaneously drop all of the Alka-Seltzer® into the water. Before dropping the Alka-Seltzer® into the water, explain to the class that they will be viewing in a condensed form how peroxides work. They should notice how violently the Alka-Seltzer® works in the 40 volume, and how much more passively the 10 volume works.

Figure 6.5

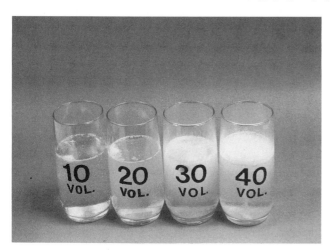

Tell the class to notice that although the various volumes of peroxide work at different intensities, they all finish at the same time.

CHAPTER 7

Using Cloth to Measure Hair Color

There is an excellent way of measuring the effect of hair color without constructing natural hair swatches, using a material called test fabric. This material is used in the fabric dyeing industry to measure the effect of dyes on various fabrics available. This same material can be used to measure how a hair tint will affect naturally light hair. Or what type of fabric comes closest to matching the hair swatch that is provided by the hair-color manufacturer.

The significance of this experiment is to show the students that colors react differently on various fibers, depending on the porosity. Fibers that have no porosity, such as Orlon 75, do not stain at all from tints. Other fibers that are more porous stain in direct proportion to the degree of porosity.

USING CLOTH TO MEASURE HAIR COLOR 25

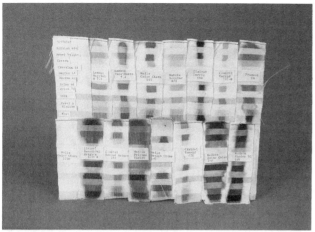

Figure 7.1

Color several pieces of material with a variety of tints from various manufacturers. Use both peroxide and non-peroxide hair colors. Compare the results of the hair colors on the material with the color chart that the hair-color manufacturer provided. We found that the wool section came closest to duplicating the manufacturer's swatches.

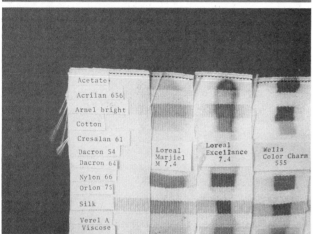

Figure 7.2

This photograph shows the variety of fabrics that are shown on the sample cloth. When experimenting with hair color on very porous hair, it was concluded that the hair color reacted similarly to the "Arnel Bright" section on the cloth sample.

PART 2

Physiological Aspects of Hair Color

CHAPTER 8

Using Your Thumbnail to Describe How Hair Color Works

The props in this manual range from complex to simple. None are as simple as using your thumbnail to describe the nature of hair color. In order to describe to your class how hair color works using the thumbnail, the thumbnail used must be free of nail polish and any type of acrylic substance.

The thumbnail is the perfect prop to describe to the class how hair color is reflected through the cuticle to the surface of the hair. Begin this class by describing how the hair is constructed. Explain that the fingernail is made up of the same materials as the cuticle of the hair. Point to the free edge of the nail; explain that the hair cuticle is the same color as the free edge of the nail. Explain that the hair gets its color not from the cuticle layer but from the melanin that is located directly below the cuticle layer. Now direct attention back to the thumbnail. Explain that only those without fingernail polish will be able to participate in this experiment.

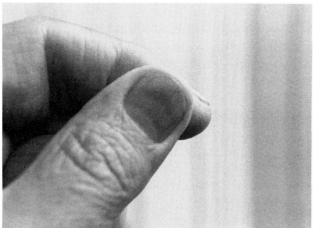

Figure 8.1

Push your forefinger up against your thumb, so that the pads of your thumb and forefinger are together. Now roll your forefinger back and forth across your thumb.

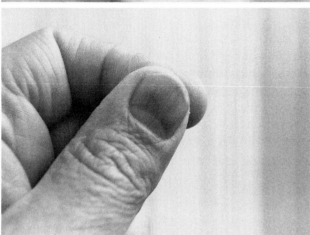

Figure 8.2

As you do this, notice how the colors directly under the thumbnail change, from crimson red to a light cream color. This is not the fingernail changing color; this is the flesh and tissue underneath the fingernail.

As the class carries out the same experiment, explain to them that when you remove color from the hair the colors being removed are located directly below the hair cuticle. The color is deposited primarily on the cuticle of the hair. It must be remembered that the cuticle, unlike the thumbnail, is in small pieces, which allows it to flex and bend. This also allows the cuticle to hold more hair color when it is deposited on the hair.

Students should understand that what you get when you apply hair color to the hair is a combination of the color that is deposited on the cuticle of the hair and the remaining color that is left under the cuticle. Remind them that when they do not wear gloves the fingernail becomes stained, just as the cuticle does.

This experiment can be further reinforced by taking some natural dark hair and scraping some cuticle off the hair. Use a sharp razor and scrape against the growth of the cuticle. The students will see that although the hair is dark the cuticle that is scraped off the hair is the same color as the free edge of the fingernail. Now very carefully scrape off some of the fingernail and compare the color of each; they are the same. Now scrape some cuticle off some hair that is tinted dark; you will see that the cuticle that is scraped off is dark. This will reinforce to your students that the tint is deposited on the cuticle, and it is not bypassed, as many would have you believe.

CHAPTER 9

Cuticle Construction

This prop should be used with the slinky hair strand (Chapter 13). Even after you explain to your students how the hair strand works, with the ability to stretch and contract, a mystery still exists. How does it stretch? How does it contract after you stretch the hair? How does the cuticle open and close? Questions fly from these wonderful, curious minds. Anyone who has taught knows the expression of glee on the faces of those who have just unraveled a mystery. This prop will elicit that expression of glee. You will have, by using this prop, explained the mystery of the construction of the hair cuticle.

CUTICLE CONSTRUCTION 31

Figure 9.1

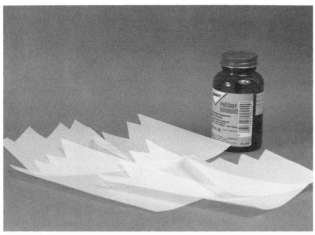

The materials needed to construct this prop are pieces of translucent plastic. Cut the pieces into 4-in. strips. Then cut one end of each strip into jagged patterns to simulate the edges of a cuticle. The strips should be cut into a variety of lengths, from short to long.

Figure 9.2

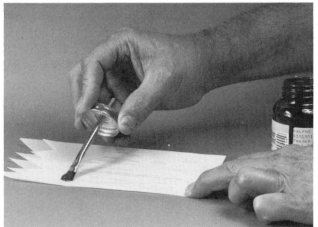

Lay the longest piece on a flat surface and apply a generous amount of rubber cement. Lay the second longest piece over the rubber cement.

Figure 9.3

Continue the process with the remaining pieces of plastic, ending with the shortest.

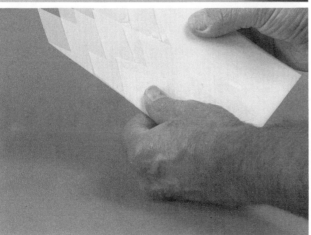

Figure 9.4

When it is completed, you will have a series of jagged pieces of plastic material adhered together with rubber cement. It is important that this prop be made just prior to your class. In order to demonstrate the elasticity of the hair, the rubber cement must remain wet. Holding the prop as shown in the photo you can move the cuticle back and forth, simulating how the hair expands and contracts.

CHAPTER 9

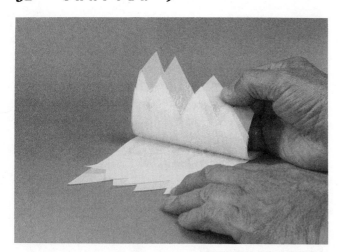

Figure 9.5

Once you show students how the hair strand expands and contracts, you can explain how the hair is constructed. Separate the pieces of cuticle, showing the rubber cement. Explain that the cuticle layers of the hair are held together by a substance that looks and acts like rubber cement.

By using this prop to demonstrate the elasticity of the hair you can easily show your students the importance of keeping hair in good condition by using moisturizers. At this point in the demonstration you explain how and why curling irons, blow dryers, perms, and hair color can cause the rubber cement to dry out, leaving hair without the proper degree of elasticity.

Chapter 10

The Giant Hair Strand

Giving the students the opportunity to see and feel what a hair strand looks like in an enlarged state opens the door to learning. It is like watching a football game from the upper deck of the stadium and having the person next to you offer you the opportunity to look through his binoculars. After viewing the game in an enlarged state through the binoculars, it is difficult to go back and view the game without them. You feel like you are missing something. I promise that if your students have the opportunity to view the giant hair strand they will have a new-found respect for this wonderful fiber.

The giant hair strand can be used for many things. For hair coloring, it will be easier to see where and how the color is deposited. For permanent waving, it will show how the cuticle is lifted from the solutions. For conditioning, it will show the difference between a strong, healthy cuticle and a damaged cuticle. You will find your students fascinated by the appearance of the giant hair strand. They will easily be able to relate to it, especially because of the numerous photographs that are currently available of enlarged views of the hair strand.

To build the giant hair strand is relatively simple, although it does require some patience. The time and effort put into this project will reap many rewards for the instructor who takes the time to build it. In many cases you will find that your students will want to build one for themselves. Indeed it can be a valuable tool for illustrating to clients the ramifications of not properly conditioning the hair. It tends to give the practitioner a greater degree of credibility. It is a bit like having a doctor use an anatomical model to explain a physical problem to you.

CHAPTER 10

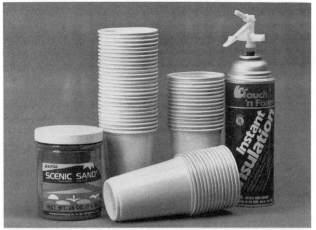

Figure 10.1
Materials needed for this project are plastic cups, sand, and foam. The foam may be purchased at a hardware store. It is used to do patching and to do small insulating jobs. The cups become the cuticle, so avoid using cups with ridges. The sand becomes the melanin, but you can also use small beads or dried rice, millet, or pasta. Sand happens to come closest to what the size of the melanin would be if the hair were enlarged to that size.

Figure 10.2
Cut tops and bottoms off the cups using an up-and-down motion with the scissors. Don't be distressed if the plastic cup tears while you are cutting; it adds to the effect.

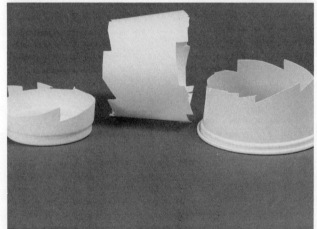

Figure 10.3
When the cup is cut into three pieces it should look like this. Be sure to save all of the pieces; they will be used in other projects.

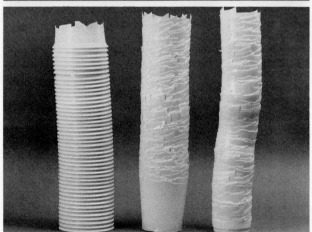

Figure 10.4
When all of the cups are cut the stacks should look something like the ones shown here. For this project we will be using the center stack of cups. You may elect to construct a longer strand. If so, you need more cups.

THE GIANT HAIR STRAND   35

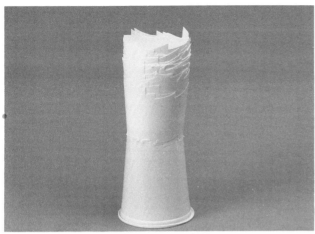

Figure 10.5
Place a portion of the stack of cups onto one of the uncut cups. This will form a seal so that the foam will not spill out.

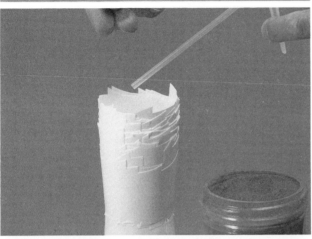

Figure 10.6
Place the long nozzle on the can of foam and squirt the foam down to the bottom of the stack of cups. The application of sand at this point is optional. It is only necessary if you plan to cut out portions from the center of the giant strand.

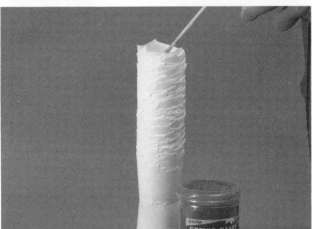

Figure 10.7
Continue stacking the cups and adding foam. If you choose, you may continue adding sand to the foam.

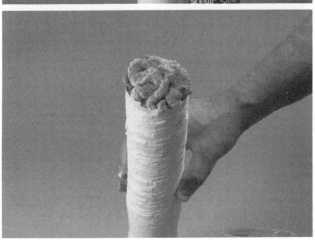

Figure 10.8
When you reach the top of the stack, fill with foam generously. Pat the stack of cups gently to make certain that the foam is compacted and all of the spaces are filled.

36 CHAPTER 10

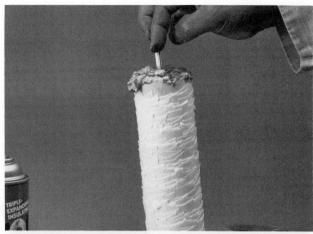

Figure 10.9
Place a short straw down the center of the stack of cups. The straw will act as the medulla of the strand. Allow the foam to dry overnight. Be certain that the stack of cups are in an upright position while the foam is drying.

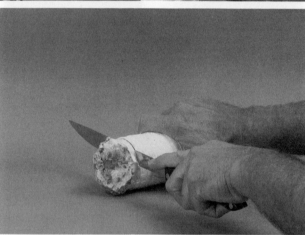

Figure 10.10
When the foam has hardened cut off the end of the giant hair strand with a sharp knife. A knife with a serrated edge works best. Use a sawing action to remove the end in order to get a clean edge.

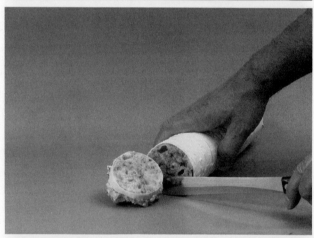

Figure 10.11
Once the end is cut off you will notice that there are spaces in the foam at the end of the giant hair strand. These are impossible to avoid.

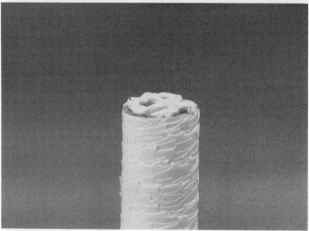

Figure 10.12
Add some extra foam to the end of the giant hair strand to fill the spaces.

THE GIANT HAIR STRAND   37

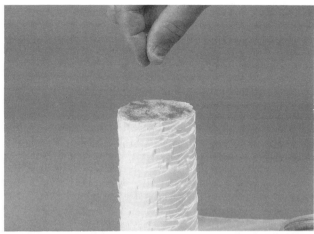

Figure 10.13

After smoothing the foam down into the crevices sprinkle some sand over the end of the hair strand to simulate the presence of melanin. The amount of sand that you use will be your choice. You may elect to use a large amount on one side of the hair strand to simulate dark hair. Then sprinkle a small amount on the other side to simulate a light strand.

Figure 10.14

Place a piece of waxed paper on top of the strand and smooth, allowing the excess foam to spill over the sides.

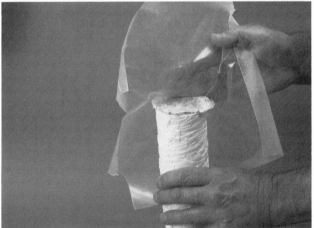

Figure 10.15

After allowing the foam to dry overnight remove the waxed paper and trim off the excess foam. Remembering where the straw was placed for the medulla, clear the foam away with the tip of the knife. Repeat the steps shown in Figures 10.10 to 10.15 for the bottom section of the strand. You may not wish to put the finishing touches on the bottom of the strand.

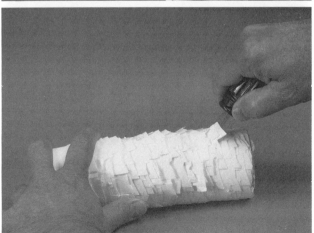

Figure 10.16

With a screwdriver force up some of the cuticle so that it simulates hair that has been damaged through chemicals. It is often said that the cuticle opens and closes, but in fact it does not. Once the cuticle is open it stays open. All that we as cosmetologists can do is to fill the cuticle and make it smooth.

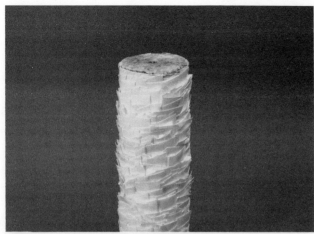

Figure 10.17

Here is the finished product showing the raised, damaged cuticle. The extent of damage that you wish to demonstrate is up to you. You may want to show much more serious damage to the hair. To do this simply raise the cuticle layer even more severely.

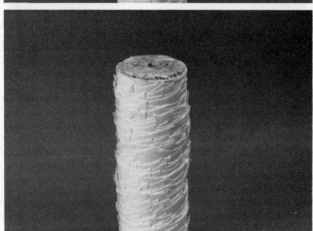

Figure 10.18

This is the healthy side of the same strand. Close, compact, and reflecting light give the hair lots of sheen.

CHAPTER 11

Chocolate Chip Cookies

When you are explaining to your students the construction of the hair and the part that the melanin plays in the overall construction, it is helpful to use chocolate chip cookies as a visual aid. Tell the class that the inside of the strand is constructed much like a chocolate chip cookie. The darker the hair strand, the more chocolate chips there are. The lighter the hair the fewer chocolate chips there are.

It is important that students can relate to something that they are familiar with. (Everyone knows about chocolate chip cookies!) Explain to the students that melanin is an intricate part of the construction of the hair. The melanin is attached to the cortex of the hair. As you lighten the hair the melanin starts to disappear; where it was attached to the cortex a void is left. If you have many chocolate chips in the cortex and you remove them all with bleach, all that you will have left is crumbs.

Analogies like this make it easy to understand the construction of the hair and what occurs when the hair is bleached. When you use this prop in your class, be sure you have enough cookies for everyone. It will make it a more memorable class.

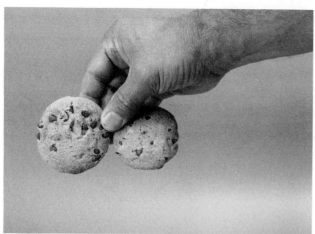

Figure 11.1

Show the class two cookies, one with many chips, simulating dark hair. The other cookie has fewer chips, simulating lighter hair.

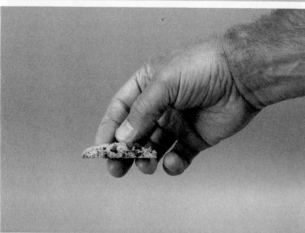

Figure 11.2

Break the cookie with the greater number of chocolate chips in half. Show the class how intricately the chips are involved in the construction of the cookie. This is how the melanin is situated in the cortex. Have them try to imagine what the cookie would be like with the chocolate chips removed.

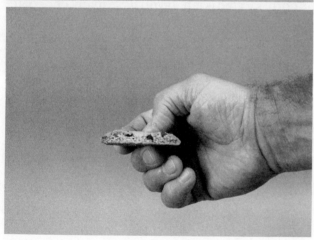

Figure 11.3

Break the cookie with fewer chocolate chips in half. Compare the two cookies. The cookie with fewer chips would represent hair that is lighter. The students will be able to imagine that if the chips were removed from the cookie with fewer chips there would still be some cookie remaining. However, there would not be much left of the cookie with many chips, representing dark hair, if the chips were removed.

CHAPTER 12

The King Crab Leg

This is a prop that you can use that doesn't take anything more than a trip to the fish market. When you go to the fish market, ask for the longest part of the king crab leg. Tell them to cut the leg in half lengthwise. That gives you enough for two classes. Store one half in the freezer for future use.

The class will understand much more about the construction of the hair if they can see a working model. The king crab is obviously not a giant hair, but the components and the proportions are similar. This will help the class understand that the inside of the hair strand is a soft, pliable, woody-looking substance, which is actually attached to the cuticle layer of the hair. The hair strand is capable of becoming very damaged if proper conditioning is not used. Sometimes it helps to cook half of the crab leg so that the class can see what the inside of the hair looks like when it has been overprocessed or abused by heating implements.

The more vivid the image of the hair strand, the better the student understands the process of coloring the hair. It is extremely important that students understand the damaging effects that can take place when coloring the hair. Only then can they prevent damage and keep the hair healthy. This prop will also help them to better understand hair construction.

CHAPTER 12

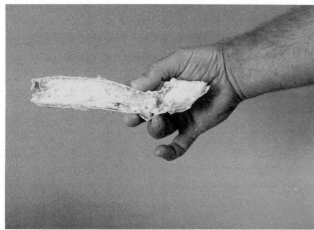

Figure 12.1

Demonstrate to the class by pushing on the inside layers of the strand that the cortex is soft and pliable in healthy hair. Show that the outside layers are made of a tough, hard, horny substance that protects the inner layer. Use this prop in conjunction with the slinky and giant hair strand props when explaining the composition of the hair.

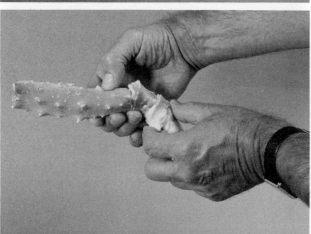

Figure 12.2

Next turn the crab leg. Demonstrate how the joint of the crab leg is constructed. Bend it back and forth, and explain that the hair is constructed in much the same way and is held together with much the same type of substance.

Chapter 13
The Slinky Hair Strand

It is difficult for cosmetology students to visualize how a strand expands and contracts. For them, the hair is no more than a fiber, a piece of thread, a strand of wire, or a blade of grass. They must be shown that the hair is a unique fiber, that it is constructed so that it will stretch and contract. To actually see this happening is to create awareness of how unique the hair strand actually is.

CHAPTER 13

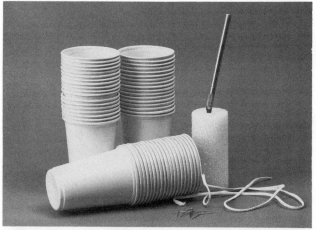

Figure 13.1
The materials required to build this hair strand are plastic cups, elastic for holding the sections together and allowing it to stretch, and straight pins to prevent the sections from sliding together. Other tools that you will need are scissors, a piece of round Styrofoam, and an Exacto knife. You may want to use foam to apply to the open end of the strand to give it a finished look. Although this last step is not necessary, it gives the strand a more realistic appearance.

Figure 13.2
Using scissors, cut the cups into three sections. Use a zigzag motion with the scissors when cutting to achieve a jagged edge; this gives a more realistic look to the finished prop.

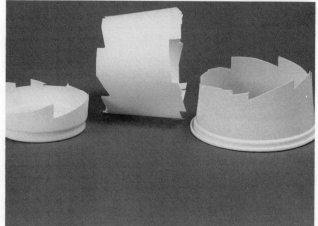

Figure 13.3
When completed you will have the top portion, the center portion, and the bottom portion. Leave the sections jagged so that the edge resembles the look of a jagged cuticle. Each of these sections will be used for building other props, so don't discard any of them.

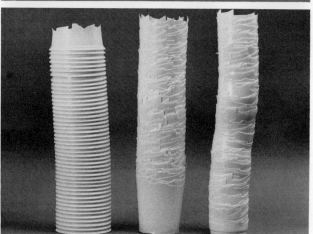

Figure 13.4
Continue cutting the cups one at a time until you have cut enough cups to give you a nice stack of each. Do not attempt to make a hair strand that is too short. It will look disproportionate and not as realistic. You need enough length so that the prop will be long enough to form a loop and still have some length left over.

THE SLINKY HAIR STRAND 45

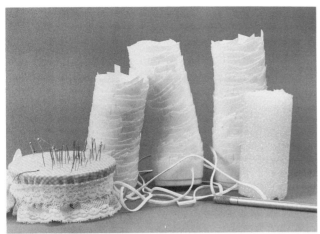

Figure 13.5
Once all of the cups have been cut, gather all of the necessary tools and parts for assembly: cup bottoms, Styrofoam, knife, elastic, and pins. If you choose to fill the ends with foam you will also need foam, sand, and waxed paper.

Figure 13.6
One at a time, place the cup bottom on the piece of Styrofoam and puncture. Any number of tools can be used for completing this procedure. In the photograph we are using an Exacto knife. The pointed end of scissors, a penknife, or a chisel may also be used. Be cautious that the puncture is not too large. Try to get the puncture as close to the center of the cup bottom as possible. Often the plastic is thickest at the center, so it will require some extra effort to puncture. If you puncture the cup bottoms on the side, the strand will not stretch equally when demonstrating elasticity.

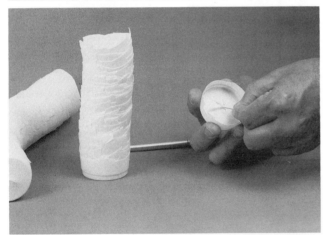

Figure 13.7
Starting at the open end, place the piece of elastic through the bottom of the cup. This inside portion will be the open end of the strand. If the strand was real, this would be the end of the hair.

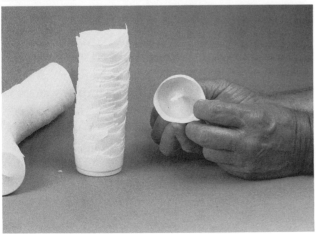

Figure 13.8
Stick a straight pin through the elastic so that the elastic will not slip back through the cup bottom.

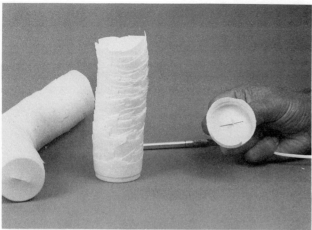

Figure 13.9
The pin should be positioned so that when the elastic is tugged on from the bottom the pin holds the elastic in place.

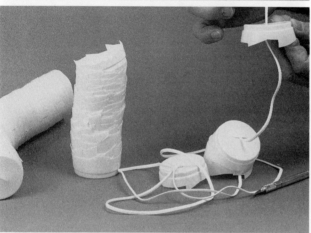

Figure 13.10
Thread the cup bottoms from the open end of each cup to the first cup bottom that has been secured.

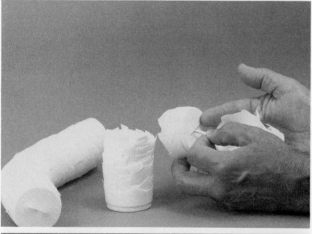

Figure 13.11
With the bottom snugged up against the first cup, place a pin through the elastic, holding the cup in place. The elastic should not be stretched before pinning. Gently tug on the elastic, release it, and then pin it. If the elastic is stretched too much you will not be able to demonstrate elasticity.

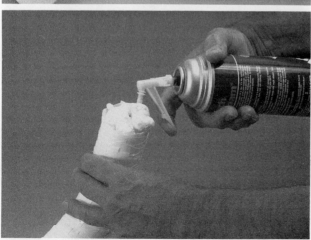

Figure 13.12
Continue this procedure until you have enough cups in place to demonstrate elasticity. Fill the end with a foam substance for a finished look. Use enough foam to fill any empty spaces at the end of the cup. Remember that the foam swells, so be cautious.

THE SLINKY HAIR STRAND 47

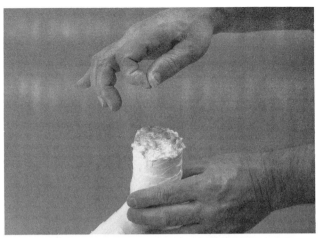

Figure 13.13
Practice sprinkling some sand onto the foam so that you can see the effect. It will aid you in determining just how much sand is necessary for the final touch.

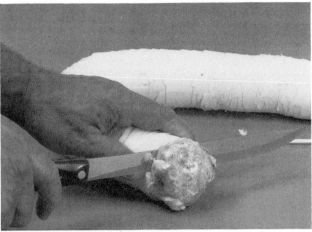

Figure 13.14
When the foam is dry, cut off the end with a sharp knife. A serrated knife is helpful in making a clean edge.

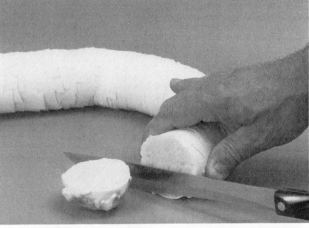

Figure 13.15
When the end of the foam has been cut off you will see some empty spaces.

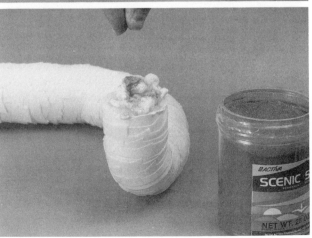

Figure 13.16
To eliminate the empty spaces in the foam and make the strand look more realistic, squirt a small amount of foam into the end of the cup. Sprinkle some sand onto the foam. The sand simulates melanin.

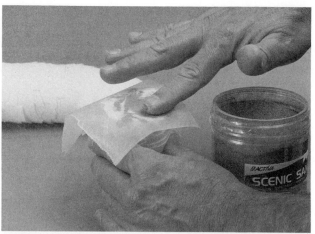

Figure 13.17
Place a small piece of waxed paper over the foam and press gently. Make the surface as smooth and even as possible.

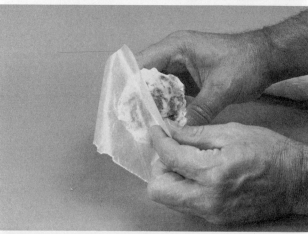

Figure 13.18
After the foam has dried, peel off the waxed paper. You will notice that the foam has spilled over slightly. This can be trimmed off with a sharp knife.

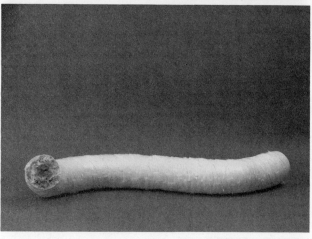

Figure 13.19
Your hair strand is now finished and ready to use in demonstrations.

This prop can be used to demonstrate to your students what happens to the hair when it is stretched. When hair is stretched, the cuticle layer becomes displaced, then returns to its original form. When hair loses its elasticity it is limp and unresponsive. The strand can be bent in circles to show that when hair is permed, the cuticle layer is displaced by wrapping the hair around a rod. When a solution is applied to hair in that position it forms a permanent curl. When you are instructing in cosmetology you will find many creative uses for your slinky hair strand.

Chapter 14
The Giant Melanin

The mystery that surrounds the decolorizing process can easily be unraveled with the use of a giant model melanin. It is a good idea to build two of these giant melanin models, one that shows light hair and one that shows dark hair. Each will have different portions of color based on the stages of lightening that the hair goes through. When the student observes the giant melanin sliced in half they can understand why the hair goes through the colors that it does. Knowing that most things dissolve from the outside, it is easy to relate to why, when one layer disappears, the remaining color can be observed.

50 CHAPTER 14

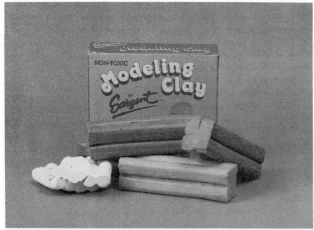

Figure 14.1
To build this prop you will need clay from a hobby or craft store. Make certain that the package of clay you purchase has all of the essential colors. The colors needed are white, yellow, orange, red, blue, and brown.

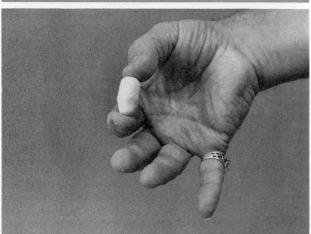

Figure 14.2
You can make a very large melanin model or one that is very small. Naturally the larger you make the melanin, the more clay is required. Here we are going to make a large melanin model to represent dark hair. We are going to start with a small white center. The white clay that we don't use for the dark hair will be used to make the light hair melanin.

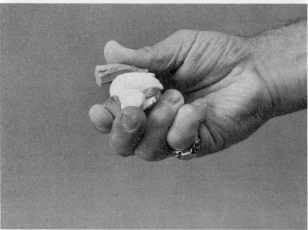

Figure 14.3
The next color that we will use is pale yellow. The yellow that comes in the package is too bright, so we will mix it with some of the white to make a pale yellow. This requires doing a lot of kneading to mix the colors. It helps to heat the clay slightly to make it soft.

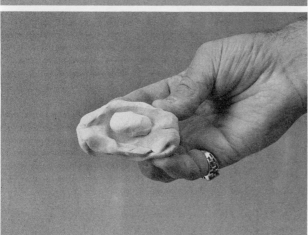

Figure 14.4
When the clay is mixed to your satisfaction, place the small white piece of clay into the flattened-out piece of pale yellow clay. Surround the small white piece of clay with the pale yellow piece of clay.

THE GIANT MELANIN 51

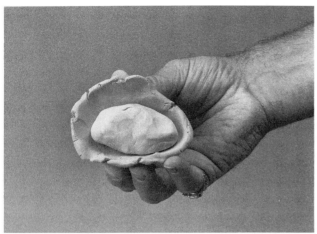

Figure 14.5

Flatten out some of the bright yellow clay and wrap this around the pale yellow clay. It is not necessary to include all of the colors that the hair would go through to become blonde. Explain to the students that the colors are reflective, like colored glass.

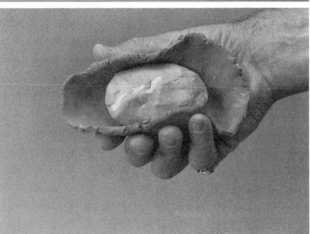

Figure 14.6

Next we will mix some of the yellow and some of the orange to produce a gold stage. A rather generous proportion of this color may be used. Try to establish the thickness of the color based on the time it would take to remove that stage from the hair when actually bleaching the hair. Wrap the gold as you did on the previous colors.

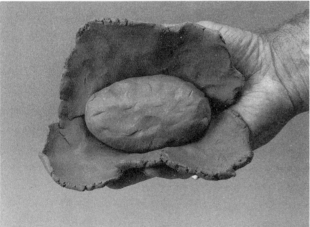

Figure 14.7

Next use orange, then red-orange, then red, then blue, then a very light coating of brown. The brown coating makes the melanin look more realistic. Rather than use the brown as you did the other colors, just knead a little color onto the surface. The students need to understand that, regardless of the color of the hair, the blue color is always the first to go. Naturally, the smaller the piece in the center that you start with, the smaller the melanin will end up.

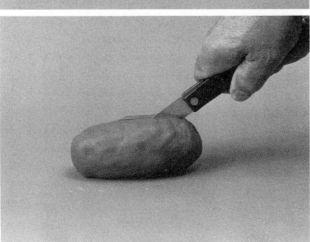

Figure 14.8

When the melanin is completed, slice it in half. Use a sharp carving knife and gently push the knife through the melanin. Do not use a sawing action. A sawing action would cause the colors to run into each other.

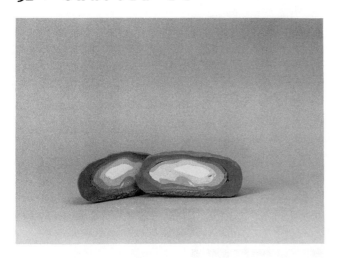

Figure 14.9

Here you see the melanin completed. Once you have shown the melanin to your class, place the two sides together. To preserve the condition of your giant melanin, place it in a plastic bag with a few drops of water. When you want to reuse the melanin, remove it from the plastic bag and slice it open again. It is particularly effective to cut the melanin open again in front of the class.

CHAPTER 15

Dissolving Melanin in the Cortex

This prop is helpful for visualizing the cataclysmic action that takes place when hair is being bleached.

54 CHAPTER 15

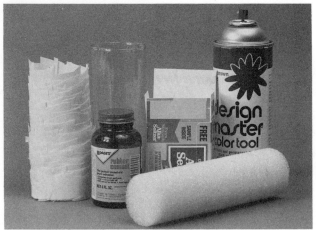

Figure 15.1
The materials needed to perform this demonstration are a tall drinking glass, a round piece of Styrofoam, Alka-Seltzer®, spray paint, and the simulated cuticle that was made in the previous class.

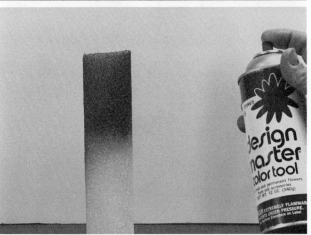

Figure 15.2
First spray paint the Styrofoam a darker color. Do not coat the Styrofoam too heavily with paint on the first coat. The spray paint has the capacity to melt the Styrofoam.

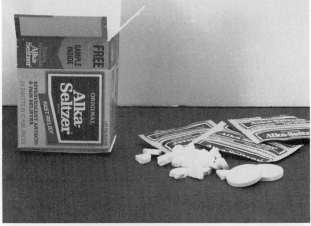

Figure 15.3
Break up a number of Alka-Seltzer® tablets into quarters. The larger the section of Styrofoam that you use the more pieces of Alka-Seltzer® you will need. You may now proceed in one of two methods, depending on the desired final effect.

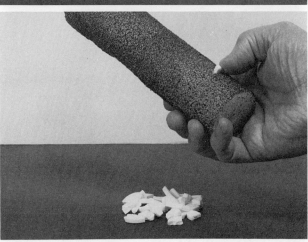

Figure 15.4
Stick the Alka-Seltzer® directly into the Styrofoam. The number of Alka-Seltzer® sections that are placed depends on how dramatic an effect you wish to create. If you want to have the Alka-Seltzer® dissolve slowly, coat it with heated wax prior to sticking it into the Styrofoam. This technique will require about five minutes for the Alka-Seltzer® to dissolve.

DISSOLVING MELANIN IN THE CORTEX 55

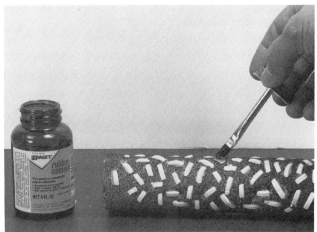

Figure 15.5

Coat the Alka-Seltzer® with rubber cement. This will slow down the dissolving process. Additional coats of rubber cement can be used to further retard the dissolving process.

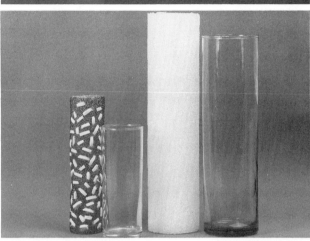

Figure 15.6

Here you see the simulated cortex finished, ready to be placed into a glass. Depending on the size of your class, you may elect to use a larger piece of Styrofoam and glass than is shown here.

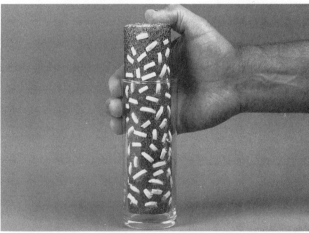

Figure 15.7

Place the Styrofoam into a glass, and force it to the bottom.

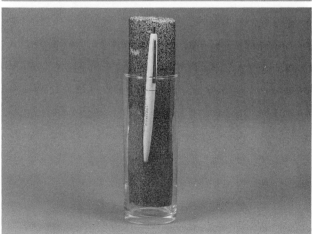

Figure 15.8

Stick an object in the back of the glass to hold the piece of Styrofoam intact in the glass. It would be very anticlimactic when you pour water into the glass to have the Styrofoam float out of the glass.

56 CHAPTER 15

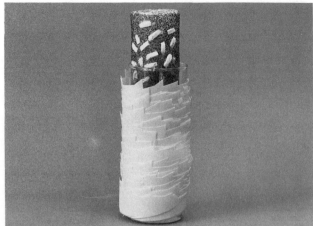

Figure 15.9
Place the simulated cuticle around the glass prior to pouring the water inside the glass. The commentary for the demonstration should sound something like "Here we have a strand of hair. We are now going to bleach the hair so that you can see what happens on the inside." At that point you peel the cuticle off, exposing the glass.

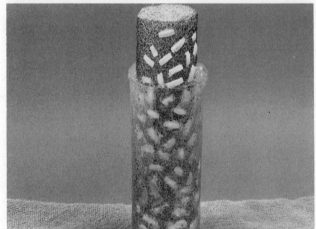

Figure 15.10
Pour water into the glass and have the class observe the chemical reaction of the melanin reacting to the peroxide. At this point explain to the class that if the cuticle was in place, the chemical reaction would be forcing its way through the cuticle layers of the hair, creating damage.

Figure 15.11
The rubber cement slows the process down only slightly. With this technique you would explain prior to pouring in the water that this is the reaction when you bleach the hair quickly. Refer to the cuticle layer that you peeled off, and explain that all of the bubbles that you see would have to find their way through the cuticle layer.

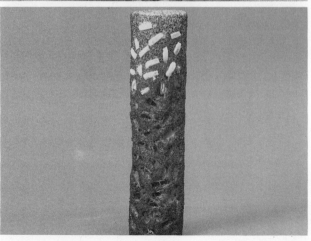

Figure 15.12
After all of the chemical action has subsided, remove the Styrofoam from the glass and allow the class to view how the hair has become weakened with the melanin no longer intact.

This is a very dramatic demonstration, which the class will remember. Another way this demonstration can be used is to have two demonstrations going on at the same time. In one glass you would have many Alka-Seltzer® tablets implanted to simulate dark hair. In the other glass you could have fewer Alka-Seltzer® tablets, simulating lighter hair. The purpose of this demonstration is to show how much weaker the hair becomes depending on the amount of melanin that is removed from the hair.

CHAPTER 16
Bleaching Dissolving Melanin

Of all the misinformation that circulates through the industry involving hair color, none is more harmful than the premise that faster is better. In the arena of bleaching (or hair lightening, as many refer to it), the condition of the hair varies tremendously, depending on the speed at which it is bleached. This prop is designed to show how important it is to bleach the hair slowly. This prop is to be used with the prop "Dissolving Melanin in the Cortex," and the graph "Bleaching Slow Versus Fast." When making this presentation you should have both the prop and the graph present.

Figure 16.1

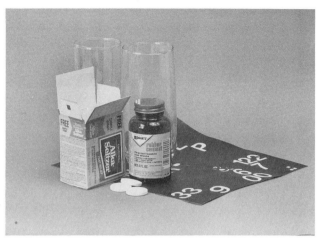

The materials needed to conduct this demonstration are: two tall drinking glasses, Alka-Seltzer®, stick-on letters, and rubber cement.

Figure 16.2

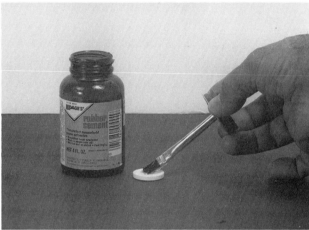

Preparing this prop is relatively simple. Take an ordinary Alka-Seltzer® tablet and cover it with rubber cement. Allow to dry, and cover with another coat. Do this on the evening prior to doing the demonstration so that the cement will be thoroughly dry. The purpose of the coating is to inhibit the flow of water to the Alka-Seltzer® so that it dissolves more slowly. Numerous other substances can be used for this purpose, such as wax, clay, chewing gum, or even paint. Whatever substance you use, be sure to test it first so that when you use the prop for the class the Alka-Seltzer® doesn't float to the top of the glass. This could ruin the demonstration.

Figure 16.3

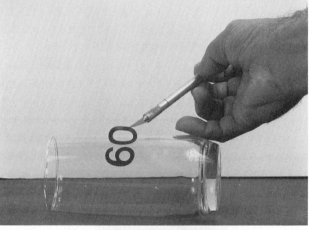

Place stick-on numbers on the two glasses. The numbers will represent the strength of peroxide in each glass. The spread of the strength of the peroxides used is entirely up to the instructor. The highest number is the highest strength that you would recommend using.

Figure 16.4

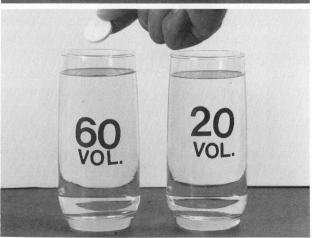

Fill both glasses with water. (We are just simulating peroxide; do not actually use peroxide.) Place the coated Alka-Seltzer® in the glass with the smaller number. Into the glass with the larger number place the uncoated Alka-Seltzer®.

60 CHAPTER 16

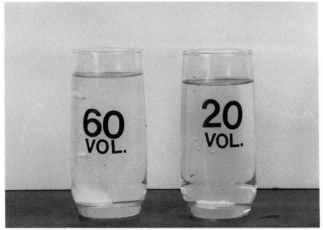

Figure 16.5
The class watches intently while the bubbles make their way to the top of the glass. When you place the uncoated Alka-Seltzer® into the glass, you describe the action as though it were a cataclysmic event.

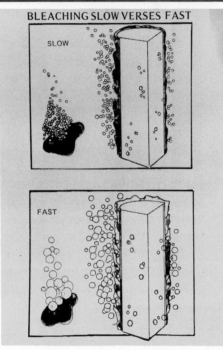

Figure 16.6
At this point show the graph while discussing the chemical reaction and how the small bubbles work their way through the cuticle. When you bleach the hair quickly the chemical action that takes place tears and shreds the hair cuticle, leaving the hair weak and splintered. Describe the lasting detrimental effect fast bleaching has on the hair.

When doing this demonstration I will often refer to an experience that I had while in the service. As part of my training I was required to learn how to fight fires. An oil fire would be started in a small compartment to simulate being aboard ship. In a few minutes the fire would be blazing. A team would have to enter the compartment to fight the fire. We wore breathing apparatus to keep the smoke out of our eyes and to allow us to breathe clean air. In those days the breathing apparatus that we wore had limited capabilities. It had a canister in the front that hung from the mask. It was about the size of a can of soup. It would last an average of 15 minutes, depending on the degree of smoke you were breathing. You could tell that the canister was losing its effectiveness when you started to smell smoke.

At that point, you would have to exit the compartment to change the canister. Then you would turn the fire hose over to a new team. This routine continued until the fire was extinguished.

The reason that I tell this story is that the chief in charge recognized that we were all very young and would probably not heed his warning about how to dispose of the used-up canisters. So he wisely went a step further. After he lectured us on how to dispose of the used canister, he took us outside. There he gathered us into a large circle, about 50 yards in diameter. He went to the center of the circle, where there was a bucket that contained oily water. "This," he explained, "is what will happen if you throw your used canister into oily water." We waited intently, staring at the bucket. As he threw the can in, an explosion of water shot up out of the bucket. At that point we were all believers. You could be guaranteed that we would dispose of our canisters properly.

I am sure that everyone remembers when they had to be shown something to believe it. After seeing it, a lasting impression was left. Sometimes a story is enough. However, when the condition of a client's hair is involved, it is important for the student to see the visual impact of bleaching firsthand.

Chapter 17

Wrap-Around Cuticle

(To Be Used in Conjunction with the "Dissolving Melanin in the Cortex" Prop)

This prop has limited usage. Its basic function is to enhance the demonstration of what happens to the cortex of the strand when the melanin is dissolved. In any of these demonstrations the more realistic you can make them, and the more students can imagine what is occurring, the more meaningful the experience will be. It is therefore important that all of the components be there. The usage of this prop is thoroughly documented in the chapter "Dissolving Melanin in the Cortex." We will therefore only deal with the preparation of this prop and not on how it is used.

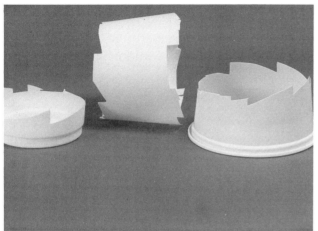

Figure 17.1

The sections of this prop are made from plastic drinking cups that have been cut into three pieces.

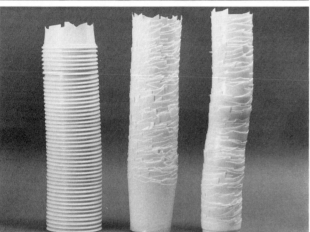

Figure 17.2

The center portion of the cup will be used to construct this prop.

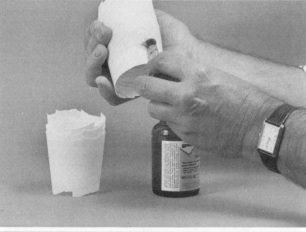

Figure 17.3

Paint a light coating of rubber cement completely around the cup. A band of rubber cement about 1 in. wide is enough to hold the cups in place.

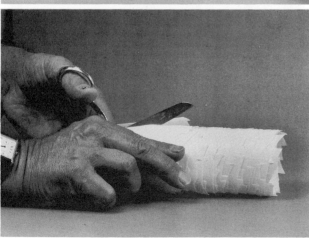

Figure 17.4

Allow the glue to dry in place overnight. This is important. If you try to cut the cups before they are dry they will warp. With heavy-duty scissors cut the simulated cuticle from one end to the other.

64 CHAPTER 17

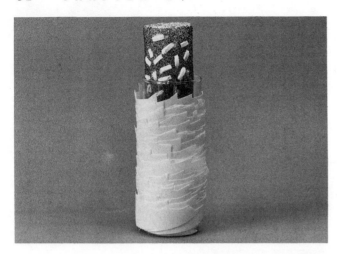

Figure 17.5
Here you see the wrap-around cuticle in place ready to be used for demonstration.

CHAPTER 18

The Decolorization Process

The decolorization process of a hair strand can be a confusing issue for a student of cosmetology. The more you can clarify this, the clearer the picture becomes.

This prop is used with an overhead projector. It is made with gels (the type used for stage lighting) and a piece of foam-core cardboard. The purpose of this prop is to demonstrate how the hair decolorizes, what colors are removed and what colors remain. It is yet another method of demonstrating that hidden beneath the cool natural color an abundance of warm tones are ready to emerge the moment you begin to lighten it.

You could make one prop for each of the natural hair color categories. I personally feel that this is unnecessary. If you describe what occurs with the other hair colors students should understand.

The gels may be purchased at stores that sell art equipment, or they may be found at a photo store if there is no stage lighting equipment store in your neighborhood. You might ask the high-school drama coach where he or she purchases the gels used in plays. Many of the stores have a booklet of sample colors from which to select. They come in different densities. Use gels with the least density for the best results.

CHAPTER 18

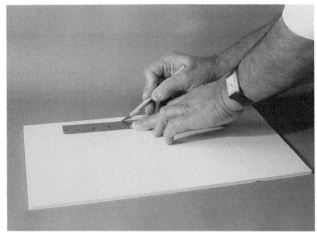

Figure 18.1
Select a piece of foam-core cardboard. The piece of cardboard should be large enough to cover the lighted portion of the overhead projector. Decide where the gels are to lie. The size of this opening can vary. I would suggest making it as large as the overhead will allow.

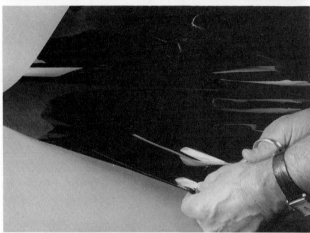

Figure 18.2
Cut the pieces of gel to fit over the opening. Make certain that gels are cut slightly larger than the opening.

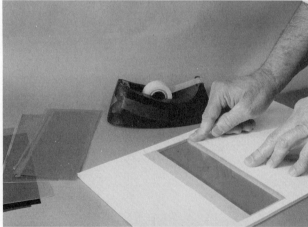

Figure 18.3
Use yellow, pink, and blue gels to complete the project. The yellow will make gold. The pink will make red, and the blue colors will tone down the red.

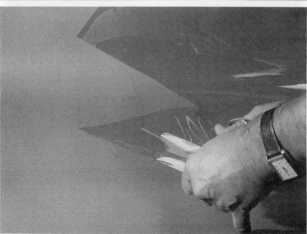

Figure 18.4
Starting with the yellow, attach the gel to the side of the opening as close as possible to the opening.

THE DECOLORIZATION PROCESS 67

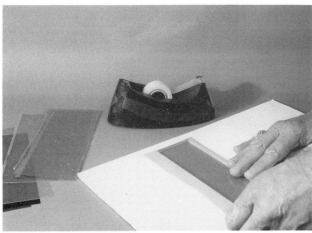

Figure 18.5
Continue attaching the gels to the cardboard so that they line up.

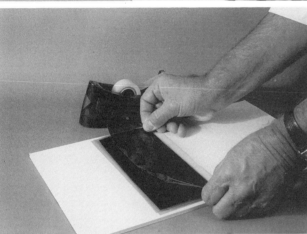

Figure 18.6
When the last gel is in place you can see how much larger it is than the first gel that was taped down.

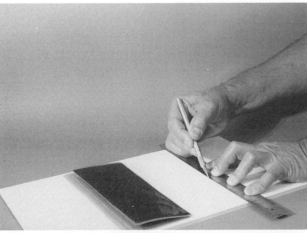

Figure 18.7
Flip all of the gels over so that the opening has nothing over it. Make a mark where the gels line up.

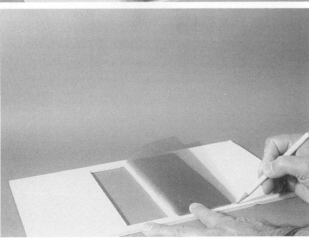

Figure 18.8
Lay out the opening where the cutout is going to be. This cutout is where the gel that has been removed is going to show.

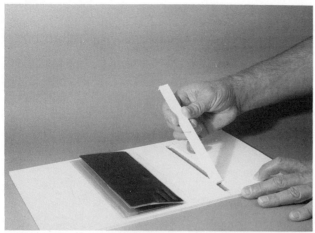

Figure 18.9
Remove the piece that has been cut out.

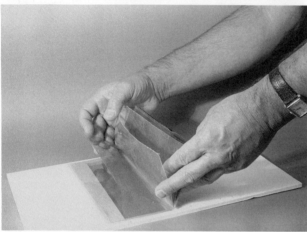

Figure 18.10
Count the number of gels to be shown. Decide on the size of the tabs that are to be cut out.

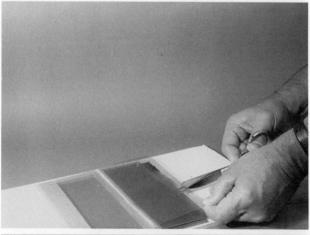

Figure 18.11
Cut the tabs out so that they overlap slightly. The tabs should be graduated in such a way so as to show the color as it is removed from the large opening.

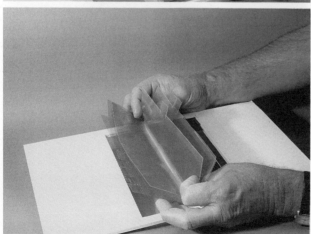

Figure 18.12
Here the prop is completed with the tabs cut. Use this prop in conjunction with the category chart that comes closest to the decolorizing process in this prop.

Chapter 19
Fast vs. Slow Bleaching

This prop is designed to show the student the tremendous difference between bleaching hair fast and bleaching hair slowly. To reinforce this fact we have taken the hair that has been bleached slowly and permed it to show that even after perming the hair it remains in much better condition than hair that has been bleached fast.

Before starting this prop, please refer to Chapter 25 on making swatches for experiments.

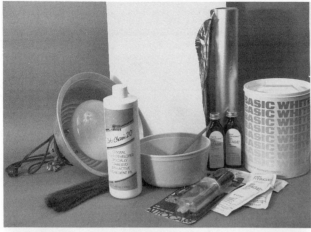

Figure 19.1

To prepare this prop you will need the following items: peroxide (20 volume and 130 volume), heat lamp, epoxy glue, mixing bowl and brush, off-the-scalp powder bleach, mild on-the-scalp creme bleach, activators, aluminum foil, prepared swatches, foam core cardboard, and black plastic stick-on letters.

Figure 19.2

Mix a mild on-the-scalp bleach with 20 volume peroxide. Make certain that all of the activators are dissolved before adding the creme bleach. Undissolved activators create "hot spots" on the hair and may weaken the hair where the undissolved activator sits.

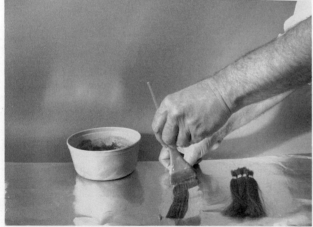

Figure 19.3

Apply the creme bleach to the hair swatches, making certain they are completely saturated. It will take about 1 hour and 45 minutes to bleach dark brown hair to a soft shade. Seven swatches of hair will be used to demonstrate this bleaching process. One extra swatch may also be used to demonstrate the slow bleaching process on permed hair.

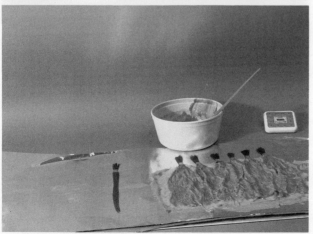

Figure 19.4

When all of the swatches using the slow process have been saturated, set the timer for 15 minutes. If the swatches that you will be processing longer start to dry out you will have to resaturate with more bleach. You may find that over the entire bleaching time you may have to mix a fresh batch of bleach.

FAST VS. SLOW BLEACHING

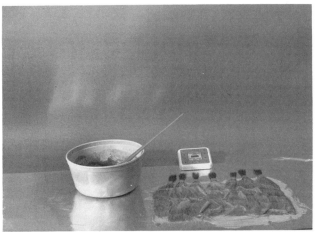

Figure 19.5

After fifteen minutes has elapsed shampoo the first swatch and set it aside. Mark the time so that when the swatches are mounted you have a record of the amount of time each swatch has been bleached.

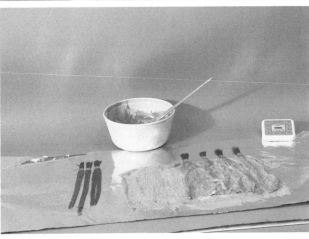

Figure 19.6

Continue this process of shampooing the bleach off each swatch as it makes a visible color change. The processing times for the swatches will be approximately 15 minutes, 25 minutes, 35 minutes, 55 minutes, 1 hour and 15 minutes, 1 hour and 30 minutes, and 1 hour and 45 minutes.

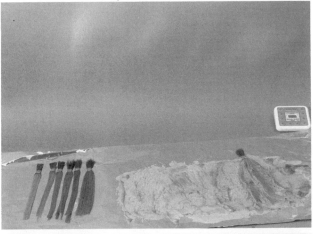

Figure 19.7

To demonstrate the effects of the slow bleaching process on permed hair, process two swatches for 1 hour and 45 minutes and perm one. The permed swatch will further demonstrate the health of the hair after the slow bleaching process.

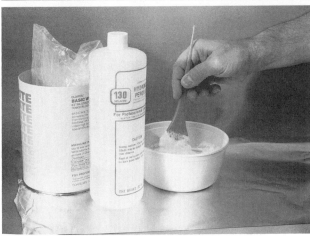

Figure 19.8

Mix a powdered bleach using a 130-volume peroxide. Mix a generous amount, as you will want to apply the bleach more than once. The heat of the lamp you will use later will cause the bleach to dry out.

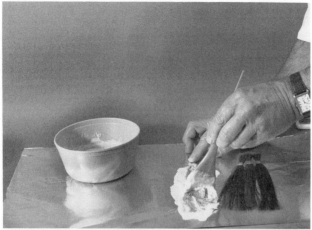

Figure 19.9

Apply the bleach generously to four swatches of hair, making certain that they are thoroughly saturated.

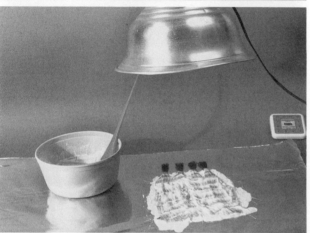

Figure 19.10

When all four of the swatches are saturated set the timer for about 30 minutes, and place the swatches under a heat lamp. With this bleach strength and heat the hair should bleach to a soft blonde shade in about 30 minutes. Remove the strands at 5, 10, 20, and 30 minutes. The faster you bleach these swatches the more dramatic the difference in condition between the slowly bleached swatches.

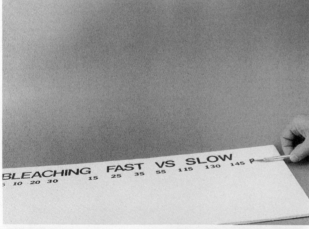

Figure 19.11

Prepare the cardboard on which the swatches will be glued. You may use any design for your prop. Be creative!

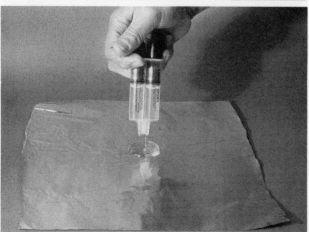

Figure 19.12

Use epoxy glue for attaching the swatches to the cardboard. The epoxy glue will assure that the prop will have a long life and the swatches will be secure.

FAST VS. SLOW BLEACHING

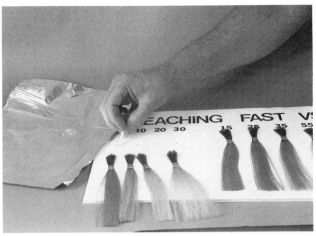

Figure 19.13
Lay out the swatches in exactly the position that you want them and make a small mark with a pencil. Take a small amount of epoxy glue and place it on the pencil mark.

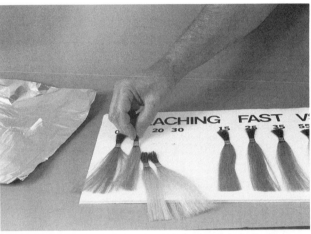

Figure 19.14
Place the swatch directly on the spot of glue, and press in place.

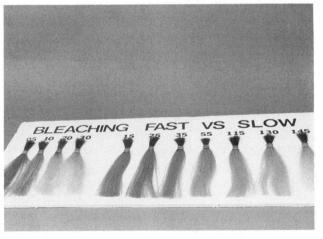

Figure 19.15
Once all of the swatches are in place allow the glue to dry. For more durability you can border the cardboard with black cloth tape.

You now have a prop for demonstrating to your students the difference between bleaching hair slowly and quickly. You can feel and see the difference. It is important for students to realize that you seldom bleach the hair just once. Bleaching the hair is an ongoing process. When the outgrowth shows, it is time to bleach the hair again. Unless you are able to keep the hair in strong, healthy condition, the client will start to experience breakage, and you will most certainly lose him or her as a client.

CHAPTER 20
How Porosity Affects Hair Color

The word *porosity* gets tossed around when teaching hair coloring as much as a volley ball does on the beach. If a color does not take as we hoped it would we say that the hair is too porous; if the color grabs on the ends we say that the hair is too porous; if the color does not take enough then we say that the hair is not porous enough. In short, we tend to blame all hair-color problems on porosity.

A definite pattern occurs when using hair coloring over porous hair. The best method of explaining to the student what happens to the hair when using peroxide colors is to show them. The word *porosity* literally means "with pores, or with voids, or openings." This, of course, would imply that the more porous the hair the more colors it will absorb. This may be true when working with non-peroxide hair colors. What generally occurs with most non-peroxide hair colors is that the hair color will work in direct proportion to how porous the hair is. The more porous the hair, the more color the hair will absorb.

This color absorption theory is true of non-peroxide hair colors. It is not true when it comes to peroxide hair colors. Peroxide makes attempting to anticipate how the hair color will respond a bit more difficult. When using non-peroxide hair colors, all you need to do is evaluate the condition of the hair by sight and feel. The degree of lightness from the natural hair color will give some indication of how porous the hair is. You may then select the hair color accordingly. Peroxide hair colors tend to absorb or reject certain primary colors depending on the porosity of the hair. The general rule is that porous hair absorbs more cool tones and rejects warm tones. Healthy hair rejects cool and absorbs warm tones. The degree to which this occurs depends on the porosity of the hair and the brand of hair color that is being used.

The chart that we are going to create here will help explain this hair-color phenomenon. If you use a chart of this type along with the accompanying graph (Degree of Porosity Based on Stage of Lightness), you may explain to your more advanced students how to anticipate what will happen when you apply peroxide to the hair. The graph assigns a number, depending on how distant the hair is from the natural hair color, which will indicate to the student how porous the hair is. The meaning of the number and how it relates to the hair condition is explained in the key. The chart does rely on some variables: whether the hair was bleached quickly or slowly, how recently the hair was bleached, how far beyond the lightest stage it was bleached, if it was permed and when. The chart is meant to be a general guideline.

Degree of Porosity Based on Stage of Lightness

STAGE OF LIFT		1	2	3	4	5	6	7	8	9	10	11	12
GROUP	1	2	2	2	2	3	3	3	3	4	4	5	5
B	2	2	2	2	2	3	3	3	3	4	4	5	
BLACK & DARK BROWN	3	2	2	2	2	3	3	3	3	4	4	5	
GROUP	1	2	2	2	2	3	3	4	4				
W	2	2	2	2	2	3	3	4					
WARM BROWN	3	2	2	2	2	3	3	4					
GROUP	1	2	2	2	2	3	3						
S	2	2	2	2	2	3							
SOFT BROWN	3	2	2	2	2								

DESCRIPTION OF DEGREES OF POROSITY

1. Compact, tight cuticle free of any chemical treatment or excessive exposure to sun or mechanical styling devices (natural hair).

2. Slightly raised cuticle, mild chemical exposure, good elasticity.

3. Moderately raised cuticle, weakness in strand, fair elasticity.

4. Excessively raised cuticle, loss of some cuticle layers, slight swelling of hair strand, poor elasticity.

5. Loss of most of the cuticle layers, excessive swelling of hair strand, lacks elasticity, slimy when wet.

Porosity of the hair as defined on the above graph has been determined by having the hair lightened for the period of time outlined on the graph for minimum bleaching times. Faster bleaching would raise the level of porosity.

The porosity will vary slightly, depending on the texture of the hair. The coarser the hair, the more porous.

If the hair is permed it will raise the porosity one full level.

If the hair is over-permed or has been permed more than once, raise the porosity two full levels.

Groups W, S, and R may also reach levels 4 and 5 porosity if continually exposed to chemical and mechanical damage or excessive exposure to the UV rays of the sun.

Non-shaded areas require special caution when perming. Level 5 on the porosity scale perm is not recommended.

NOTE: Group R, the red category of natural hair color, is not listed on graph. It falls into the same pattern as the W, warm brown category.

CHAPTER 20

To make this prop you must first refer to Chapter 25 on making swatches for experiments. The number of swatches that you use for this prop will depend on how much of a learning tool you want it to be. You can color as few as two or as many as twenty. Besides this tool showing how hair color acts on various hair strands, it also gives a general indication of overall color deposit depending on the level that is being used and the amount of lift a particular color has. The chart shown here will contain ten swatches.

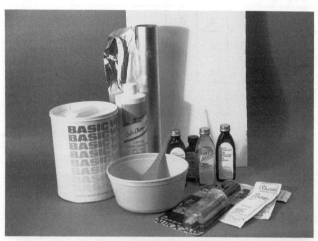

Figure 20.1

To complete this chart you will need the following materials: tint brush and bowl, peroxide, powder bleach, aluminum foil, various colors, foam-core board, stick-on letters, resin glue, creme bleach, and activators. You will also need the desired number of swatches.

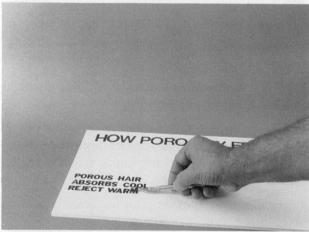

Figure 20.2

Prepare the foam-core board by adding the message that you wish to convey to your students. It is not a billboard, so keep the message to a minimum.

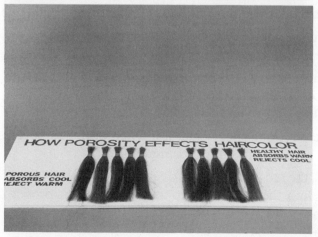

Figure 20.3

Lay out the swatches on the board to decide the number of swatches that can be comfortably used.

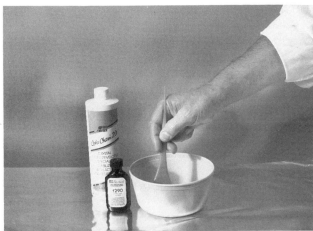

Figure 20.4

Mix the high-lift tint in a bowl. Mix according to manufacturer's instructions.

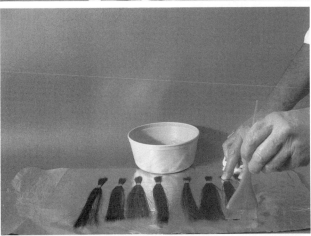

Figure 20.5

Apply the high-lift tint on the strand, making certain that it is completely saturated. Leave the hair above the crimp natural so that you will always know what the natural hair color was. Allow the strands to process for the appropriate amount of time, then shampoo off.

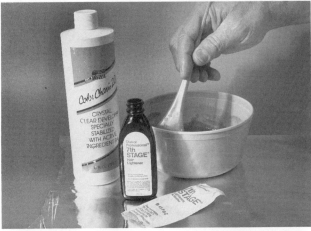

Figure 20.6

Mix some scalp bleach in a bowl. The strength of the bleach will depend on the depth of the hair that you are working on. The darker the hair, the stronger you will want the bleach to be. You will want to have a definite demarcation line between the high-lift tint and the bleach.

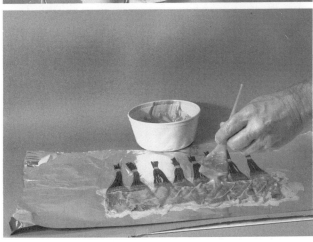

Figure 20.7

Cover two-thirds of the strand with the creme bleach. Make certain that the strand is thoroughly saturated. Apply the bleach on both sides of the strand. Allow the bleach to process until there is a well-defined demarcation line.

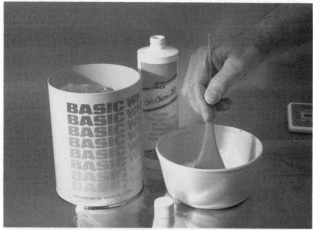

Figure 20.8

Mix some scalp bleach in a bowl. This stronger bleach will be used to create extra porous ends. You will want to bleach this hair beyond the pale yellow stage. This will most likely take more than one application of bleach.

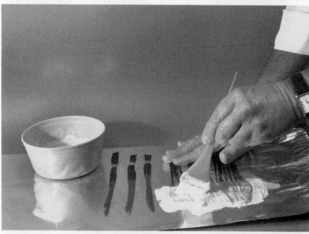

Figure 20.9

Apply the bleach to the bottom third of the strand.

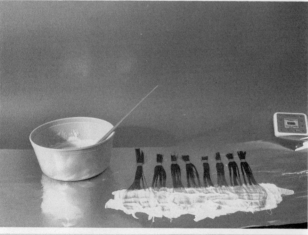

Figure 20.10

Bleach the hair for an hour. Shampoo the bleach and reapply; continue to reapply until the hair is at the palest blonde stage, almost white. When the hair has reached this stage, shampoo and dry the swatches.

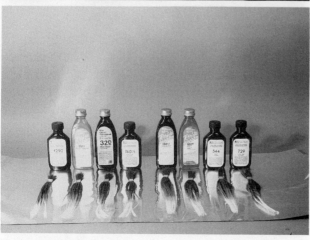

Figure 20.11

Select a number of colors to use — some light, bright reds, some neutral shades, and some cool shades. Place the swatches on a piece of aluminum foil with bottles of color directly behind each swatch.

HOW POROSITY AFFECTS HAIR COLOR

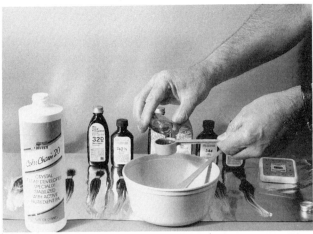

Figure 20.12

Carefully mix the colors in direct proportion to the manufacturer's instructions. Time the swatches very carefully to get an accurate rendering of the colors.

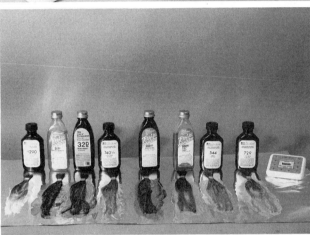

Figure 20.13

Mark the swatches on the metal crimper while the hair is processing so that they do not get mixed up.

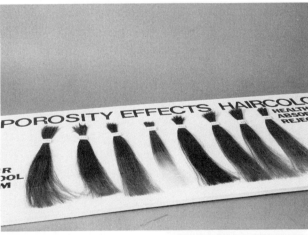

Figure 20.14

Lay out the swatches on the foam-core board that has been prepared.

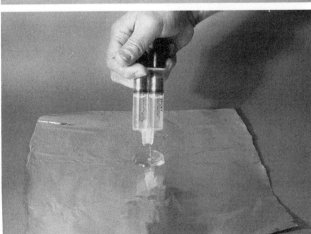

Figure 20.15

Mix some epoxy glue together to attach the swatches to the board.

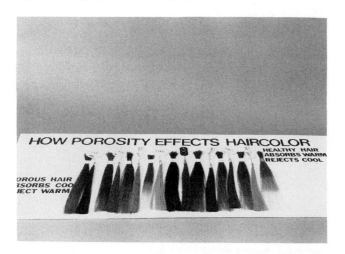

Figure 20.16
Attach the swatches to the cardboard with the epoxy glue. Place the manufacturer's swatch ring of the color next to your colored swatch ring. You will be able to see the difference in the effect of hair color, depending on the type of hair.

Chapter 21

How the Hair Reflects Color

This prop is best used to show why and how hair color changes when the hair is wet, compared to when it is dry. It can also be used to show your class the changes that occur within the hair strand when peroxide hair color is applied to the hair. Although the explanation used with this prop is rather simplistic, it offers the student a view of hair color that is easy to understand. This prop shows the hair before it is colored and what occurs after it has peroxide color applied to it. You can construct this prop in any number of ways. This is just one of them.

All of the supplies needed to prepare this prop can be found in an art store or a drafting supply store.

CHAPTER 21

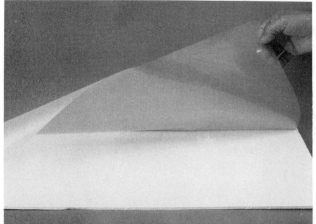

Figure 21.1
Prepare a piece of foam-core board. It should be large enough to be seen clearly by the entire class. Place a piece of clear cellophane over the foam-core board. The cellophane is the type used for doing overlays in artwork.

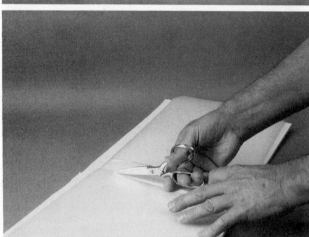

Figure 21.2
Once it is in place cut the cellophane in half. One half will be used to show a virgin hair strand; the other half will be used to show the effect after applying hair coloring. It will show the wet/dry reflection of hair coloring.

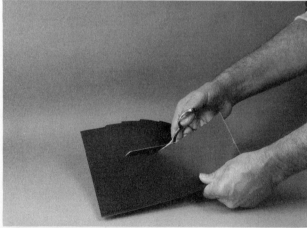

Figure 21.3
Cut a sheet of stick-on colored paper into the shape of the outside of an enlarged strand of hair. Stick-on colored paper can be purchased from an art supply store. It comes in a variety of colors of different intensity. A medium brown shade was used here.

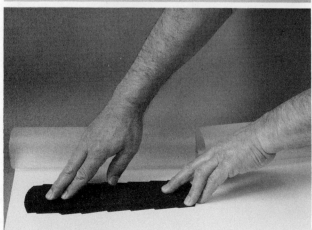

Figure 21.4
Place the cutout hair strand directly on the foam-core board. This color will indicate the color of the hair before it is colored.

HOW THE HAIR REFLECTS COLOR

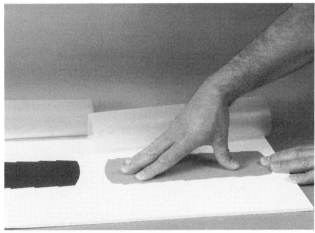

Figure 21.5
On the other side of the foam-core place a stick-on piece of a lighter colored paper in the same shape as the previous hair strand. The color that you use should be one of the stages the hair would go through in the lightening process. Here we are using an orange color.

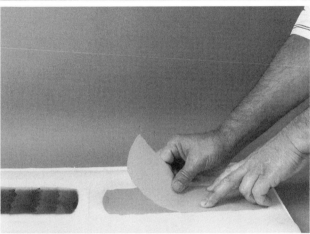

Figure 21.6
Place an even lighter yellow stick-on colored paper on top of the thick cellophane, lined up with the orange colored one. Make sure that the two pieces are identical shapes.

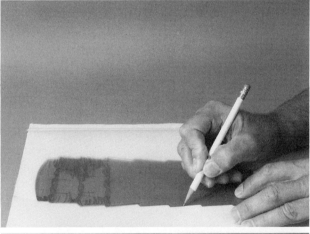

Figure 21.7
With a pencil, draw in lines and shadings that would simulate the outside of the cuticle of the hair. This is the type of cellophane that allows you to draw on the surface. Repeat this on the side that has the light yellow color as well.

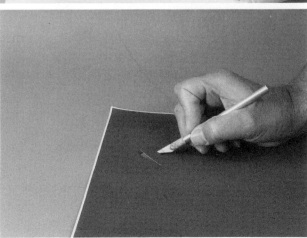

Figure 21.8
Cut out two arrows from a dark grey stick-on piece of paper. Make the two arrows the same size.

84 CHAPTER 21

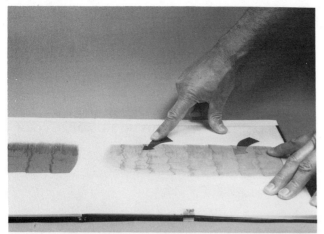

Figure 21.9
Stick the two arrows on the surface as indicated. The full arrow on the left is stuck on top of the cellophane. The arrow on the right has the top portion of the arrow on the cellophane, and the pointed part of the arrow on the foam-core board.

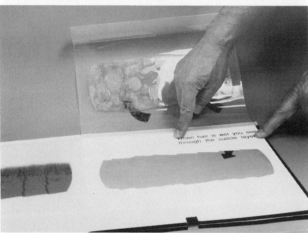

Figure 21.10
Have type set or use stick-on letters to read "When the hair is wet you see through the cuticle layer." Place these letters as indicated in the photo.

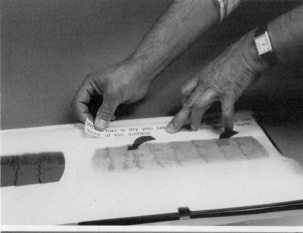

Figure 21.11
Over the cellophane to the left side of the strand place the words, "When the hair is dry you see more of the surface."

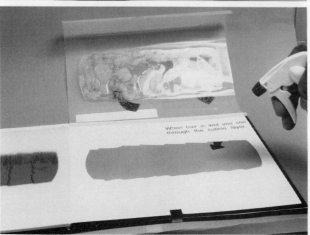

Figure 21.12
To demonstrate the intent of this prop, spray some water over the right side of the orange colored hair strand, marked "when hair is wet."

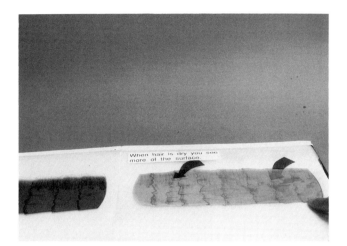

Figure 21.13

When you place the cellophane over the wet section it will show more of the orange color underneath. The side that is dry will show more of the lighter yellow color.

The purpose of this prop is to demonstrate to the student not to judge the color of the hair when it is wet. When the hair is wet the more visible color is the color of the melanin, which often is the unwanted red tones that will appear in hair. When the hair is dry, the unwanted red tone is toned down, and the color on the cuticle plays a more dominant role.

This prop may also be used to show what happens to hair when it is colored with peroxide-type hair colors. The simulated strand on the left is without color, and the surface of the cuticle is translucent, revealing the natural melanin beneath the cuticle layer. On the right it shows what occurs when the hair is colored. The color is deposited on the surface of the cuticle as well as altering the natural melanin to a lighter color. It is the combination of what is deposited on the surface of the cuticle and the altered natural pigmentation that gives the hair its final color.

PART 3

The Psychology of Hair Color

CHAPTER 22

Hair-Color Category Charts

When I think back to the early days of my career, when hair coloring was as mysterious to me as nuclear science, I ask myself "What would have helped me feel more comfortable about using hair color?" The answer is, knowing how the hair color is going to respond on a particular head of hair. This seems to be a simple enough order. However, when you consider the variety of natural hair colors, the different degrees of porosity, and the various amounts of grey found in the hair, it is not that easy to predict.

In a survey held by the International Haircolor Exchange, an organization of hair colorists, of over 300 cosmetologists, cosmetology instructors, and cosmetology students, the question was asked "What do you find most confusing about hair color?" The most frequent answer was "I don't know how the color is going to turn out when I put it on," followed closely by "I don't know what color to put on the hair to get the color I want."

The more you as a cosmetology instructor can reduce the unpredictability of a formulation, the more confident the hair-color student will become. To do this you need to build props to help show your students the decolorizing process that the hair will go through.

If we divide the world population into four natural hair-color categories, we can simplify the process of identifying natural hair color. It is extremely difficult for the hair-color student to identify natural hair coloring by simply looking at the hair under natural light. This is much too difficult to do with any degree of predictability. When speaking of hair color, or any kind of color, describing color is a very difficult thing to do. These props, along with the natural hair-color badges included in this book, will help you conduct a lively class to help the student identify natural hair coloring and how it will respond to color.

I can assure you, with a great deal of confidence, that if you follow the plan laid out in this book your students will have no difficulty in identifying natural hair coloring.

Identifying natural hair color is only part of the exercise. The other part of the exercise is attempting to describe the decolorizing stages that natural hair color goes through, depending on what color it is. The purpose of these props is to show students that all natural hair color can be broken down into four major categories. Understanding this is a major hurdle in helping your students unravel the mystery of hair coloring.

We will discuss in the next section on hair-color badges how to help the student discover the four major hair-color categories.

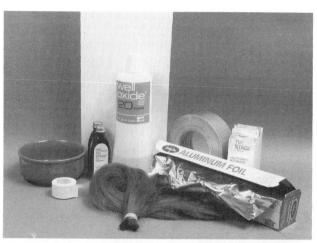

Figure 22.1

To build this prop you will need the following materials: tint brush and bowl, creme on-the-scalp bleach, aluminum foil, natural hair, duct tape, white bandage tape, peroxide, foam-core board, and black stick-on letters.

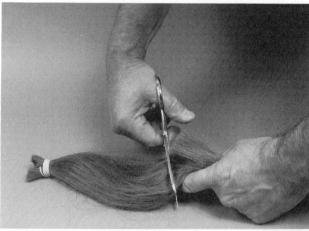

Figure 22.2

Because of the unusual length of the hair we will cut it in half. This will provide us with an abundance of hair.

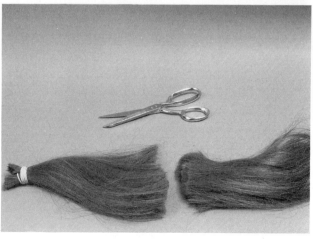

Figure 22.3

The length of the hair is still too long (about 8 in. long). We will cut it more as we proceed with this prop.

90 CHAPTER 22

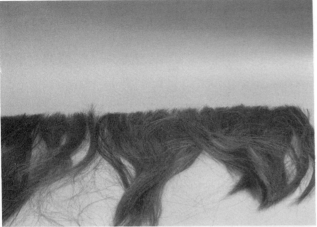

Figure 22.4
Spread the hair out, keeping the top of the hair straight. Distribute the hair as evenly as possible.

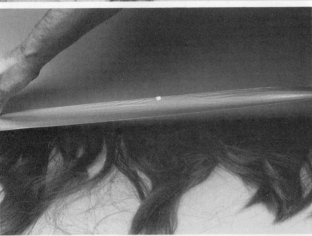

Figure 22.5
Place the duct tape down over the edge of the hair. At least half the width of the tape should overlap the hair.

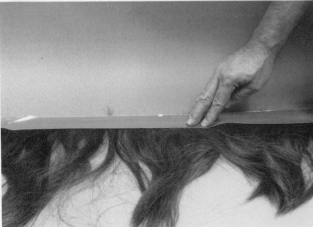

Figure 22.6
Press down firmly on the tape so that the hair adheres to it.

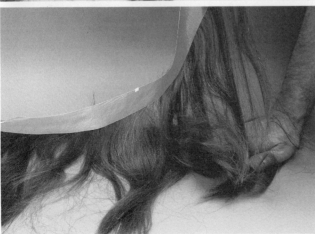

Figure 22.7
The tape will grab only the hair on the top surface. When lifting the tape, pull some of the excess hair away. The hair that is pulled away can be used for a second and third run with the tape.

HAIR-COLOR CATEGORY CHARTS 91

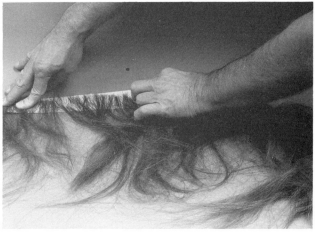

Figure 22.8

Turn the tape over and remove some of the excess hair that has not adhered to the tape. Keep the excess hair that is pulled off in an orderly stack with the ends all facing in the same direction. This hair will be used for more strips of hair.

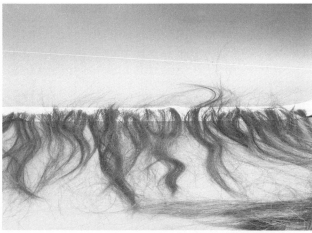

Figure 22.9

With all of the excess hair pulled away the only hair remaining will be the hair that has adhered to the tape.

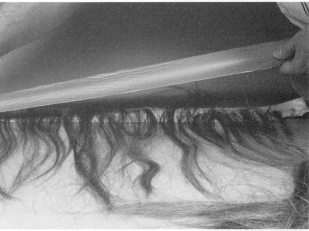

Figure 22.10

Place another piece of duct tape directly over the tape that is already in place. Line up the tape carefully with the tape that is already in place.

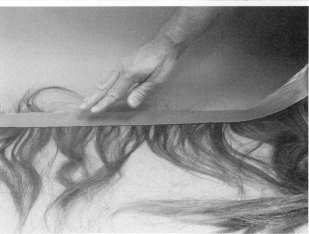

Figure 22.11

With a quick motion stick the top tape down directly over the first piece of tape.

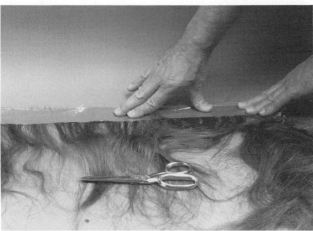

Figure 22.12

Press down firmly on the tape, making certain that the hair adheres to the tape. We now have tape on each side of the hair.

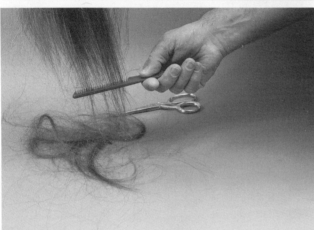

Figure 22.13

Gently comb the excess hair out of the strip of hair. The hair that is removed is discarded. Do not attempt to save this hair for future use.

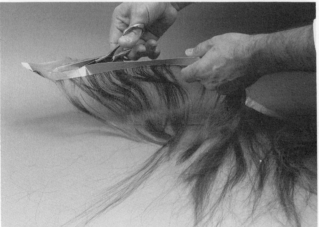

Figure 22.14

Cut the tape in half to minimize the amount of tape attached to the hair.

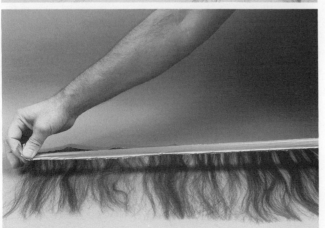

Figure 22.15

Comb the strip of hair as straight and smooth as possible. Because of the length of the hair it is possible to make two strips of hair. Tear a piece of duct tape lengthwise and carefully line up the strip of tape so that it is halfway between the first section of tape and the ends of the hair.

HAIR-COLOR CATEGORY CHARTS 93

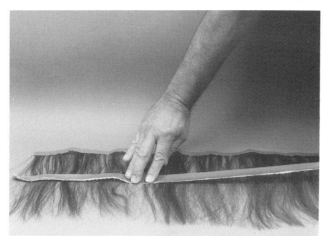

Figure 22.16

Stick the tape firmly on the hair, making certain that it adheres.

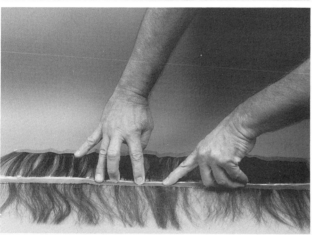

Figure 22.17

Turn the section of hair over, and place another piece of duct tape on the opposite side, lining up the tape evenly.

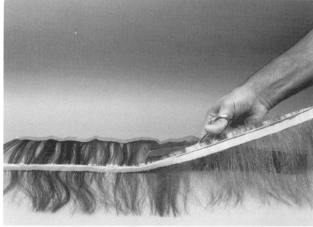

Figure 22.18

Cut the two sections apart. Cut the hair directly over the top of the lower piece of tape.

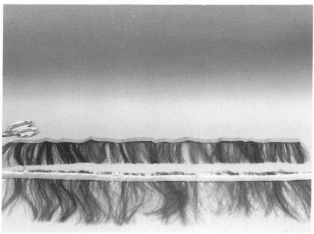

Figure 22.19

Here we see the two sections cut apart. We have managed with one section of long hair to make two shorter sections, which will better serve our needs.

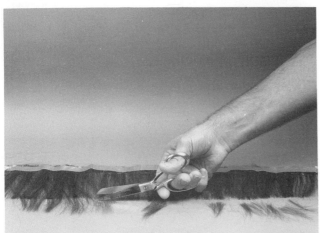

Figure 22.20
Place the section that is slightly longer on top of the shorter section and trim the ends so that the two sections are even.

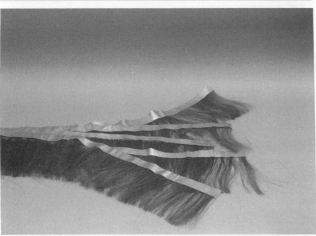

Figure 22.21
Continue this same technique until there are enough hair sections to complete all of the stages of lightening. Refer to the chart on hair-color categories to determine the number of stages the hair will go through to become blonde.

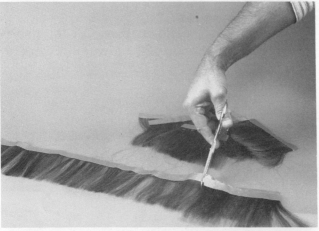

Figure 22.22
Cut the strips of hair into 6-in. sections. Save the smaller sections that may be left over at the end of the strip.

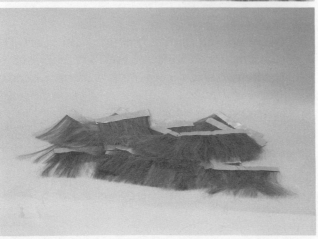

Figure 22.23
For this prop we need twenty-two sections of hair. When making and cutting these long strands, some sections will have been lightened from exposure to the sun. You may use these lighter sections to indicate the first stage of bleaching.

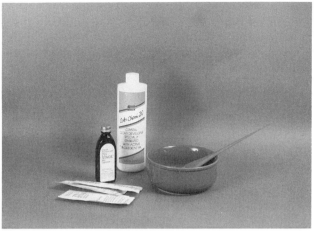

Figure 22.24

Mix up a mild on-the-scalp bleach to lighten the hair. Do not use an extremely strong bleach.

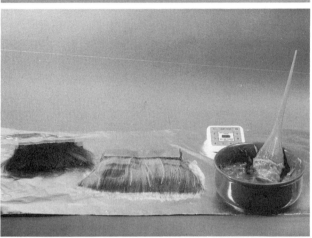

Figure 22.25

Using a tint brush, apply bleach to both sides of each of the strands until the estimated number of swatches are completely saturated. It is better to have a few extra swatches than not enough. Four natural sections should be left out. Two sections are to indicate the natural color, the other two to show the first stage of lightening.

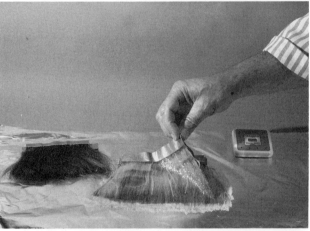

Figure 22.26

Immediately after the last sections have been saturated flip the entire stack over and peel off the first two sections that were saturated.

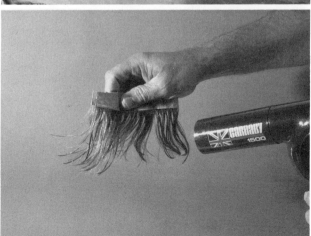

Figure 22.27

Shampoo and blow dry the hair to make certain that the section is visibly lighter than the last strands that were shampooed and dried. If it is not, resaturate the strands with bleach and allow the strands to process further.

CHAPTER 22

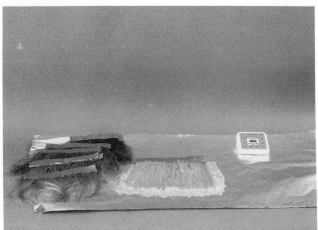

Figure 22.28

After the bleach has processed for one hour, it should be reapplied. Although the bleach continues to process it does so at a very slow pace.

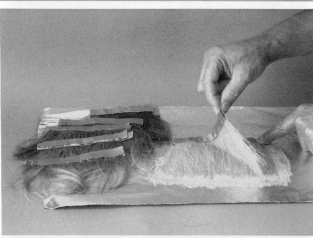

Figure 22.29

You will find that as the hair gets lighter the time span between stages increases.

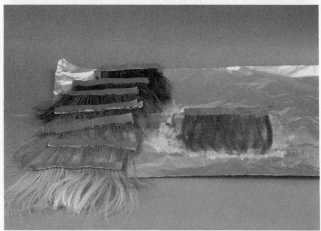

Figure 22.30

Continue this process until the last section is pale blonde. For a dramatic effect you may bleach the hair beyond pale yellow to show the damaging effect of over-bleaching.

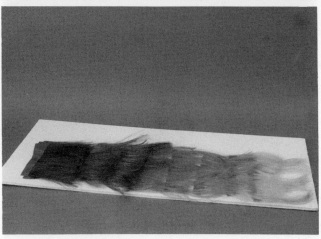

Figure 22.31

Lay out the sections of hair as they will eventually appear when the prop is completed.

HAIR-COLOR CATEGORY CHARTS 97

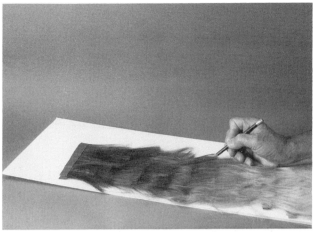

Figure 22.32
Make faint lines where the sections are to appear on the sections of foam-core cardboard.

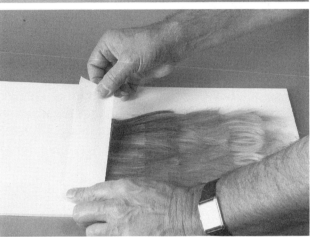

Figure 22.33
Starting at the lightest stage near the bottom of the cardboard apply each stage of hair color to the cardboard with white bandage type tape.

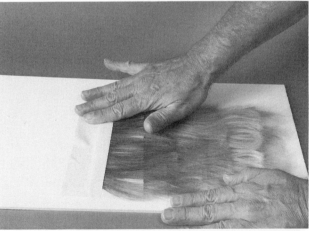

Figure 22.34
Continue working up toward the top of the cardboard, placing the strands of hair on each other in an overlapping fashion.

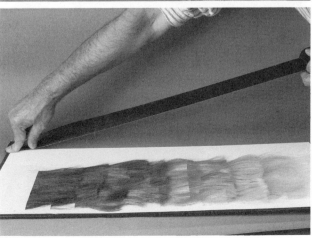

Figure 22.35
Once all of the stages of hair color are attached to the cardboard, finish off the edges with black duct tape. This will give the prop more durability and produce a framed effect.

98 CHAPTER 22

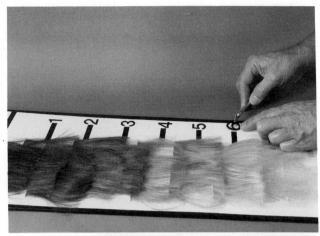

Figure 22.36
Finally, indicate the stages of lightening by placing lines next to the various shades. Next place numbers next to the lines, with the lower numbers representing the darker hair shades.

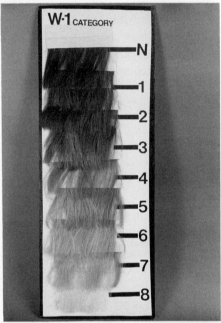

Figure 22.37
Here you see the finished prop. This prop indicates in the smallest, most visible changes, the stages of lightness this category of hair color goes through. These gradual changes are constant, and will not change regardless of the type of lightener you are using.

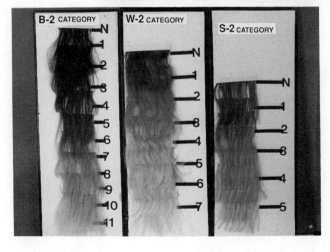

Figure 22.38
Make as many props as possible for each category of hair. Having the ability to view the differences in how each category lightens will help students predict the outcome of hair coloring.

Chapter 23

Natural Hair-Color Badges

After you have given the lecture on the various hair-color categories, have your students identify their own natural hair color. You will most often have a variety of natural hair colors in your classroom.

Prior to your lecture prepare some badges. Some examples are shown on the next page. You may feel more comfortable designing your own or having a printer design them to your specifications. You can predict, based on the area of the country, the percentage of each of the categories you will need. The basic ratio is 6 B, 2 W, 1 S, 1 R. The badges should be printed on labels that will adhere to clothing without affecting the garment.

Distribute to each student one of each category of badges. Have the students choose the badge that represents their natural hair color. Once this exercise is finished, you ask if anyone in the class is having difficulty in identifying their hair color. During this dialogue you have the opportunity to ask the types of questions that will be asked during a consultation with a client. Your students will have the opportunity to mirror your questions when they have a client in the chair whose hair they are attempting to identify. You will find that students have a very easy time identifying their own natural hair color. Next have the students check the badges on their fellow students, and allow them to have a general discussion on natural hair colors.

Once the appropriate badge has been placed on the student you can collect the excess badges and use them in future classes. Although the initial investment is substantial, you will find it is well worth it, since they help students better identify natural hair color.

CHAPTER 23

Figure 23.1

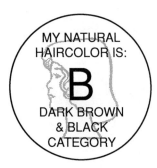

Figure 23.2

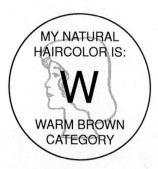

Figure 23.3

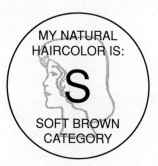

Figure 23.4

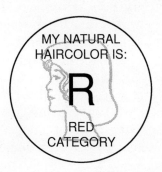

CHAPTER 24
The Consultation Book

The session when the color to be achieved is determined by both the hair colorist and the client is called the consultation. Whatever tools can help to determine the best color for a client should be used. A client who is coloring her hair for the first time will be very apprehensive. "Will I like the results? What will my friends, co-workers, and family think? If I don't like it now, what will it look like when it is growing out?" These and other questions are racing through the client's mind.

Some controversy exists about whether a manufacturer's hair-color chart should be used for consulting with a client. Exposing a client to an array of hair colors on a chart with color names listed can be a risky way to deal with a client who is making a hair-color choice. Using the hair-color chart will put the client in charge of the consultation and allow her to select her own formula from the chart.

Using the chart is often done when the colorist lacks confidence and is looking to the client for guidance. Often the client will take complete charge and dictate what colors are to be used, assuming that the color will turn out as it appears on the chart. The colorist will lose the respect of the client, who will ask to see the chart from then on to adjust the formula.

In the most successful consultations, props are not used, but the colorist describes the outcome of the color to be used. It helps for the colorist to use words that will conjure up in the client's mind the most flattering colors. Using words like creamy, warm, luscious, soft, and pale to describe the color is helpful. The colorist must paint a picture of beauty for the client to imagine. If the client is still apprehensive and needs more reassurance it helps to use someone in the salon as an example to describe how a color can be adjusted to suit your client. You would say to your client, "Something like the color Bridgett is wearing, only with slightly more highlights." If this does not work, the next step should be a photograph of different hair colors. It is best to have a photo album with photographs of an array of colors to discuss with your client. It may also work the other way around. Have your client show you how she imagines her new hair color by bringing in some photographs of a successful hair-coloring process. The following prop will help you decide what to use on your client's hair.

102 CHAPTER 24

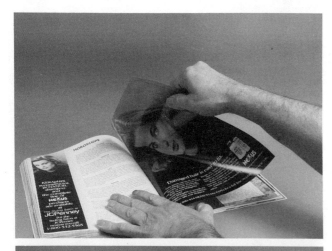

Figure 24.1
Cut pictures from magazines of a variety of hair colors. Gather pictures of both males and females. It is useful to include pictures of young children whose hair has been lightened from the sun.

Figure 24.2
Trim the pictures so that the focus will be on the hair and the face. Remove all background clutter from the pictures. When you are trimming the pictures you may find that two identical pictures have appeared in two different magazines. Before you discard one of the two pictures check them to be certain that the coloring is identical. Often the same pictures will appear to have different color variations. Use these two pictures to show the client that lighting and surroundings can make the same hair color look completely different.

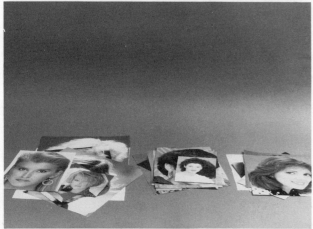

Figure 24.3
Sort the pictures into categories of blondes, redheads, and brunettes. You may choose to have subcategories of, for example, light and dark brunettes. It is also helpful to have groupings of dimensionally colored hair and examples of hair colors for men. Use as many sections and categories as you feel will offer a good variety as well as ease of using the consultation book.

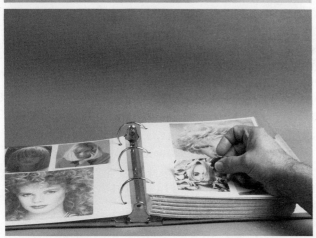

Figure 24.4
Purchase a hard-cover three-ring binder for your consultation book. The book will be used often, so make certain that you choose one that is durable. Arrange the pictures in the book as you have sorted them. You may choose to go from light to dark or to intermingle the color differences within a particular category.

You will get a lot of use out of this book. Do not make the mistake of keeping the same pictures in the book for more than one year. Even though the pictures are protected in a plastic cover, they start to look dated and should be changed.

PART 4

Creative Aspects of Hair Coloring

CHAPTER 25
Making Swatches for Experiments

Cosmetology instructors generally agree that the best way to learn hair coloring is by doing it. This does not mean that if we want to learn how a new product or a new shade will respond we should practice on our clients. We need as many clients in beauty school as in salons. Therefore it is recommended to educate students on the importance of making and using hair swatches when experimenting with hair colors. Whenever you cut off some long hair, you should save it. Try to accumulate as much hair in as many colors as you can.

I have tried many methods of making hair swatches for experimentation. The method that we will be showing here is the fastest and the neatest. I believe that it holds the hair as well as any other method of making swatches. The nice thing about this technique is that if you suddenly want to do an experiment on a strand you can make one in a couple of minutes, without waiting for the glue or fingernail polish to dry as in other methods.

Whenever you are asked a question by one of your students about hair coloring, you can encourage them to color a swatch and see for themselves. Without a swatch to look at, trying to describe a hair color is extremely difficult, if not impossible.

MAKING SWATCHES FOR EXPERIMENTS 107

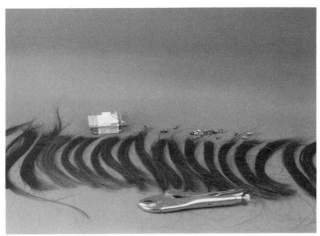

Figure 25.1

Separate the hair into swatches that are uniform in size. You will also need crimpers and a pair of vice grips to squeeze the crimpers together.

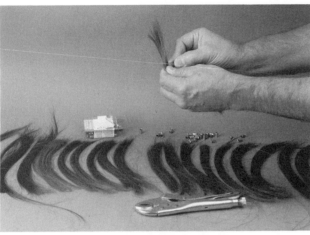

Figure 25.2

Grasp the swatch in one hand and straddle it with a bobby pin or a piece of wire.

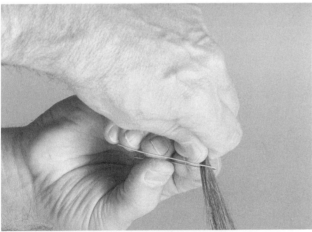

Figure 25.3

The strand should be big enough to allow the experiment to be seen, yet small enough to pass through the crimper. Crimpers come in various sizes. Pick a size about 1/8 inch.

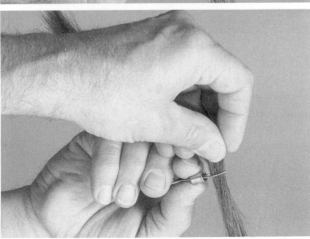

Figure 25.4

Slide one of the crimpers over the wire.

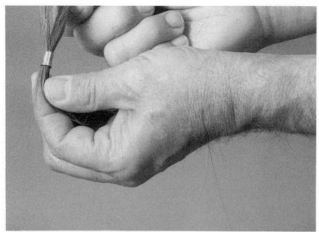

Figure 25.5

Pull the hair through the crimper. If there is too much hair to pull through the crimper, remove some of the hair.

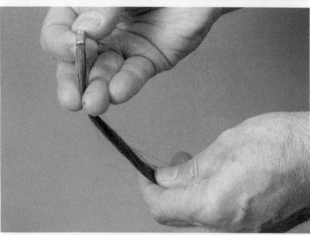

Figure 25.6

Hold the crimper near the end of the strand. Leave some hair on the opposite side of the crimper. When the strand is eventually colored the portion on the opposite side will remain natural. The student will then have a better idea of what the color of the hair was prior to the hair-color treatment.

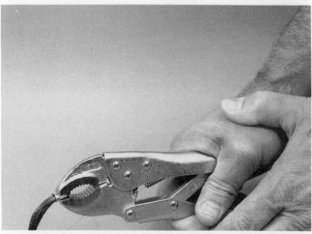

Figure 25.7

Squeeze the crimper firmly to be certain that the hair is firmly attached.

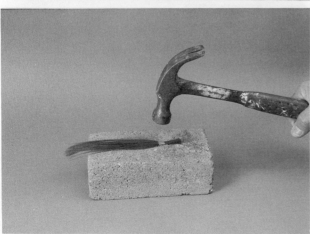

Figure 25.8

Gently tap the crimper with a hammer. This assures a firm grip on the hair. Do not strike the crimper too hard, as you could break the hair.

MAKING SWATCHES FOR EXPERIMENTS   **109**

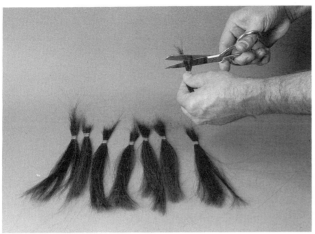

Figure 25.9
Continue steps 1 through 8 until you have the desired number of swatches made. Trim the short ends so that they are uniform.

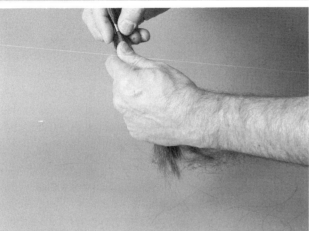

Figure 25.10
Gather up the swatches and line up evenly.

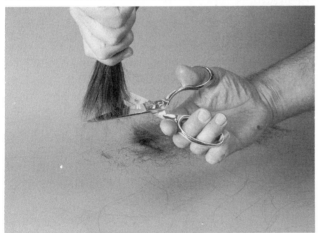

Figure 25.11
Trim the excess hair off the ends.

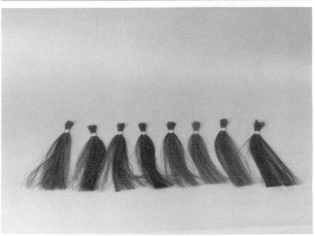

Figure 25.12
The completed swatches are now ready for your testing and excperimentation. It is never a good idea to practice on your customers. With just a little practice you will become an expert at making swatches.

CHAPTER 26

Hair-Color Chart

Of all the props, classes, and lectures, nothing furthers the overall knowledge of hair color more than having students of hair coloring make their own hair-color chart. Anyone who has gone through this time-consuming exercise knows the value of actually putting hair color on human hair and witnessing the results. Manufacturers tend to embellish and sometimes exaggerate the capacity of their hair-coloring products. This adds to some of the confusion that students experience.

I suggest that you emphasize to students the value of learning one manufacturer's line of hair color well. It becomes extremely difficult to learn and teach hair color when students are exposed to numerous lines of hair-color products. This is a weakness of many cosmetology schools.

Each manufacturer utilizes their own method of teaching with their own terminology. This makes it difficult for the student to comprehend. Hair-color teaching is so intertwined with products it is impossible to teach without relating to a product. The basic motive of the manufacturer is to sell, not to teach. If you listen to a product manufacturer give a class in hair coloring, the formulas and problem-solving techniques are given with only their line of hair coloring. This does little good if the student graduates from school and goes into a salon that does not use that particular hair color. It would be impossible and of little value for the student of hair color to learn a little bit about many hair colors. Therefore it would be in the best interest of the student to learn one line of hair coloring well first. The information gained from that experience can translate what they have learned to other lines of hair coloring.

Determining what line of hair coloring to use in a beauty school requires the same reasoning a salon uses to select what line to carry. First you determine the availability of the color (how long does it take to get it once you order it). Next you must consider the range of colors (does it have all of the colors you will need). Price, of course, is a factor when it comes to selecting a line of hair coloring (particularly for beauty schools, where the prices that can be charged are minimal). Next are support materials. Are there enough color charts so that each student may have their own? Does the manufacturer's representative stop in periodically to keep you informed of new products and concepts?

In my opinion you should have one major line of hair coloring, and one additional line to back it up and make comparisons. For instance, one hair-color line may have blonde shades with a greater degree of lift. Another line of hair color may have an overabundance of green in their brown shades. There really are no bad hair colors. It is just a matter of learning to work with the colors and understanding what they are capable of. After you have worked with a number of brands you will be able to say that they all have their own strengths (outstanding shades) and weaknesses (inferior shades), but there are many good product lines. Damage to the hair occurs when the product is misused. The product itself is not damaging.

If school owners and instructors are concerned about not being biased toward one particular line of hair color, they can change the product line periodically.

In order to stay product neutral I am going to use a fictitious line of hair coloring when showing how to build this prop. I also realize that the idea of making your own hair color is not a new, revolutionary idea. It has been done for years. By following this procedure for building a chart, you may come up with some even better ideas of how to make this procedure as simple as possible for your students.

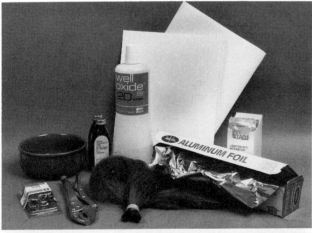

Figure 26.1

The materials needed to product this prop are human hair, preferably from the same head, aluminum foil, mixing bowl, presentation folders, scissors, Exacto knife, 20 volume peroxide, tint brush, on-the-scalp creme bleach, activators, vice grip pliers, crimp sleeves, and your choice of hair colors.

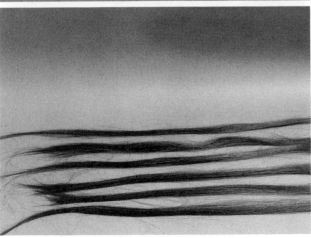

Figure 26.2

Lay the hair out in strips. Keep the sections uniform, with the cuticle all going in the same direction.

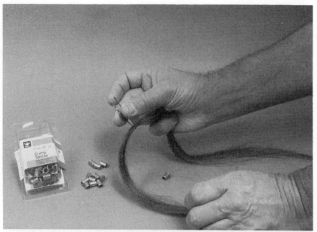

Figure 26.3

With a bobby pin or hairpin straddle the strand of hair.

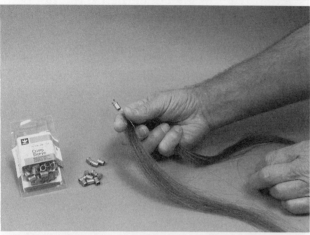

Figure 26.4

Insert the crimping sleeve over the open end of the bobby pin. If you find that there is too much hair in the strand to pull through the crimping sleeve remove some of the hair from the strand and adjust the remaining strands accordingly.

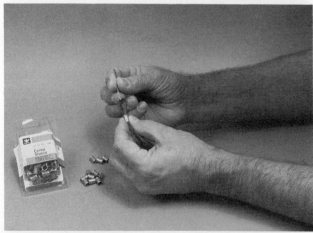

Figure 26.5

Pull the hair through the sleeve so that the crimping sleeve is only around one strand.

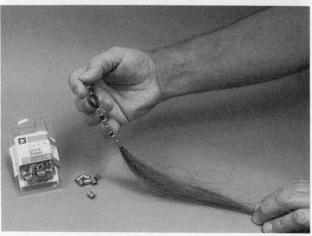

Figure 26.6

Continue this process until you have the desired number of crimping sleeves on the strand. This is determined by the length of the hair and the desired size of the swatches.

HAIR-COLOR CHART 113

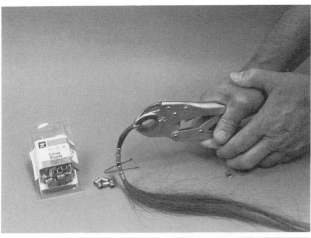

Figure 26.7

Starting at the scalp end of the strand place the crimping tool on the end of the strand and with the vice grips clamp down on the crimping sleeve, securing the hair.

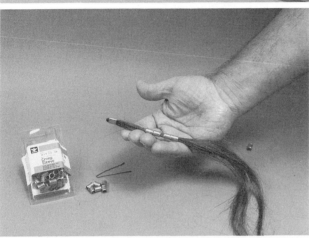

Figure 26.8

Here you see the first crimping sleeve in place.

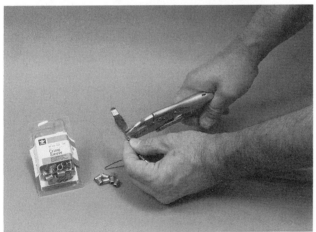

Figure 26.9

Measure down 1½ inches and secure another crimping sleeve.

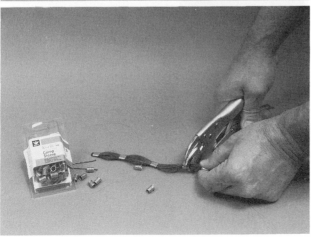

Figure 26.10

Continue placing the crimping sleeves down the strand every 1½ inches.

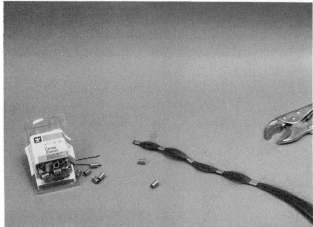

Figure 26.11

The hair will start to get thinner as you move closer to the end of the strand. When the hair starts to get noticeably thinner, stop placing the crimping sleeves. It is important that the strands are consistent in size.

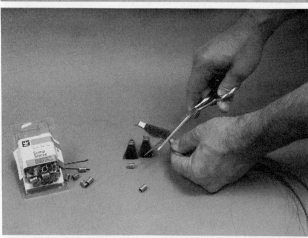

Figure 26.12

Separate the swatches by cutting the hair just above the crimping sleeve.

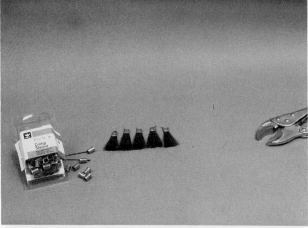

Figure 26.13

Here you see five perfectly matched hair swatches ready for coloring. Continue using this same procedure until there are enough swatches to test a variety of colors.

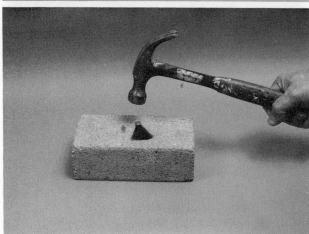

Figure 26.14

Before starting the process of lightening the swatches fatten the crimping sleeve further by tapping it with a hammer. This will assure you that the hair will not become dislodged.

HAIR-COLOR CHART 115

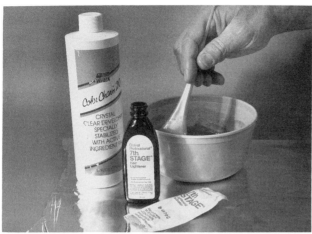

Figure 26.15

Mix an on-the-scalp bleach solution to bleach the swatches prior to applying the hair color.

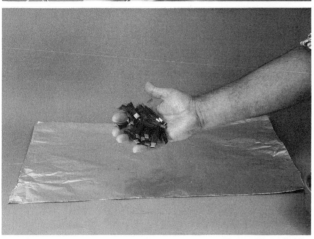

Figure 26.16

When you have completed making the proper number of swatches, gather them all up and dampen them with water.

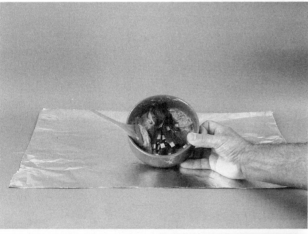

Figure 26.17

Put the swatches in a bowl containing mild on-the-scalp bleach.

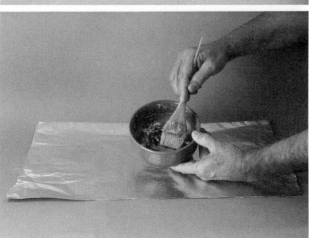

Figure 26.18

Make certain that the swatches are completely saturated with bleach. The reason for pre-bleaching the swatches is so that you can observe with greater accuracy the amount of color deposit there is in a particular shade.

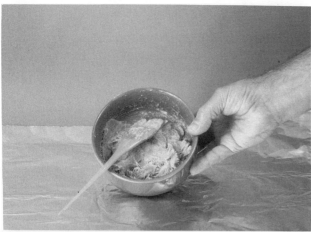

Figure 26.19

Allow the swatches to process in the bleach.

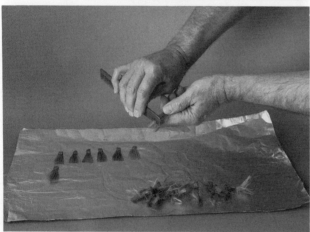

Figure 26.20

When the hair has been bleached to a yellow stage, shampoo and condition the swatches. Take the swatches one at a time, comb them smoothly, place on a piece of foil, and allow to dry.

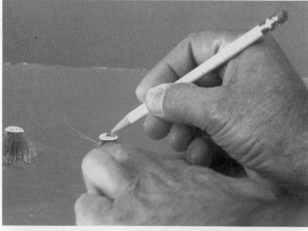

Figure 26.21

Place a small sticker on the crimping sleeve and identify the color that is going to be used on that particular swatch. Do not use ink that will run when you get it wet. Using a pencil with a #2 lead is a safe bet.

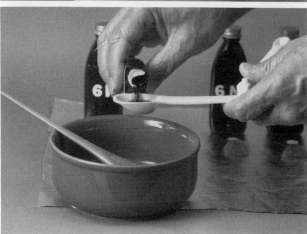

Figure 26.22

It is extremely important that the hair color that is to be placed on the swatch be mixed accurately. Measure the tint and the peroxide to the exact increments.

HAIR-COLOR CHART **117**

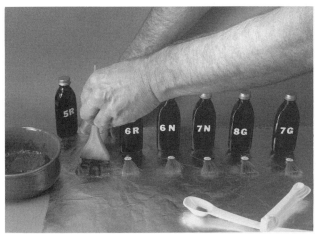

Figure 26.23
Apply the hair color thoroughly and generously to both sides of the swatch. Mark on the aluminum foil when the color is to be removed. The hair-color timing must be accurate as well. There is no sense in going to all of the effort to make a swatch card and have it be inaccurate.

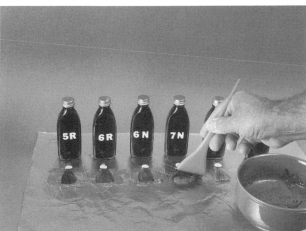

Figure 26.24
Continue this procedure until all of the swatches have been colored. When the hair color has been on the swatch the proper length of time, shampoo, condition, comb, and allow to dry. When doing this as a class project, mix all of the hair colors and have the students go from bowl to bowl coloring their swatches. Each student should have a sufficient amount of work space to process their swatches.

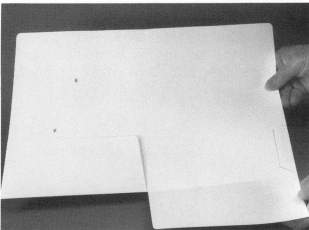

Figure 26.25
Use a standard glossy white presentation folder for the inside of the hair-color swatch chart.

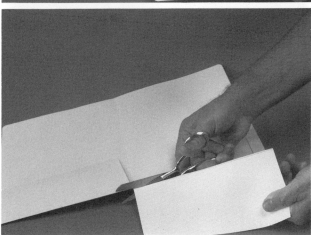

Figure 26.26
Cut the flaps off the presentation folder, leaving a heavy piece of cardboard folded accurately in half.

118 CHAPTER 26

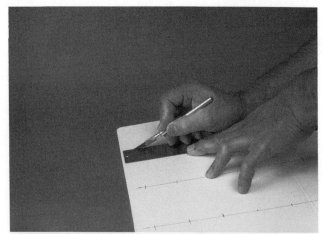

Figure 26.27
Proceed to plan the layout of swatches on the non-glossy side of the folder. The distance between each swatch will be determined by the number of swatches.

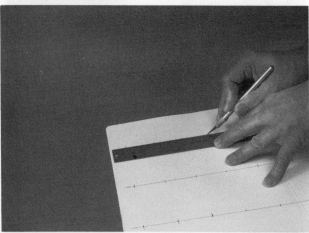

Figure 26.28
After the layout is completed, make a ½-in. cut in the cardboard where each swatch is to be placed.

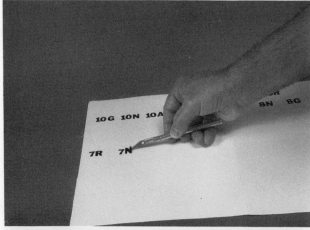

Figure 26.29
When all of the cuts have been completed flip the chart over and place the numbers and letters of the hair colors where the swatches are to be placed.

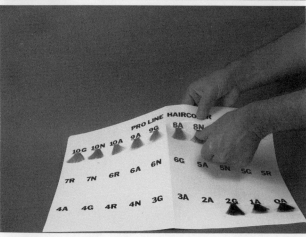

Figure 26.30
Slip the swatches into the slits. Be careful not to tear the slit when placing the swatches.

HAIR-COLOR CHART   **119**

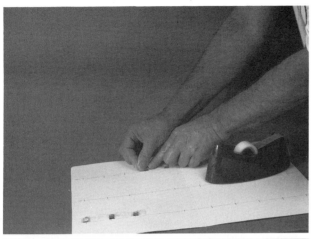

Figure 26.31

As you place a swatch flip the chart over and place a piece of tape in the back of the chart to secure it.

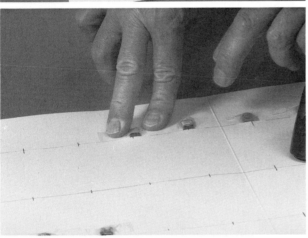

Figure 26.32

Continue this process until all of the swatches are in place.

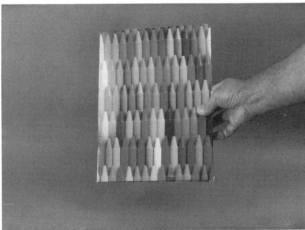

Figure 26.33

For the outside of the hair-color chart we have selected a colorful graphic of a variety of crayons.

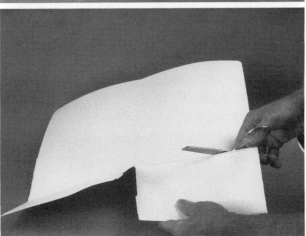

Figure 26.34

Trim off the excess flaps just as you did on the glossy white inside cover.

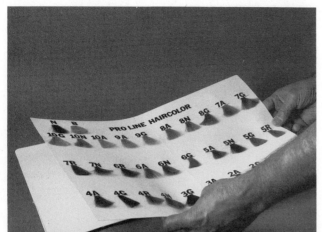

Figure 26.35

Place the inside cover with the swatches on top of the colorful outer cover to make certain that they match up.

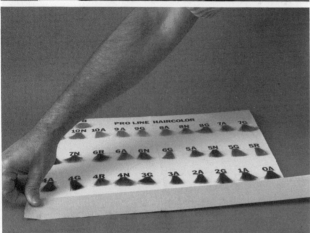

Figure 26.36

Measure some duct tape to the exact size of the folder. Using scissors, cut the tape in half.

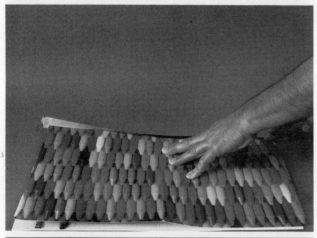

Figure 26.37

Place the tape along the edge of the chart to hold the two folders together and to give it some durability.

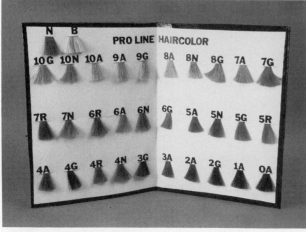

Figure 26.38

Here you see the completed chart with the swatches in place. In the upper-left corner are two swatches. One is the natural hair (N); the other indicates the stage of lightness that the hair was lightened/bleached to (B).

This color chart will give users valuable information and aid them in hair-color decisions. The color chart is especially valuable for students who end up working in a salon where little or no color work is done.

Color charts may be expanded in many ways. You may want to construct a hair-color chart to show the amount of lift that occurs at each level of hair color. This is accomplished by coloring natural hair rather than pre-bleaching.

The hair-color swatch chart is an invaluable tool that can be kept by students for years to come. It will make a student much more competent in making hair-color decisions.

CHAPTER 27

Shuffling Cards

How dimensional hair coloring can be used to solve hair-coloring problems is sometimes difficult to explain. The student who lacks hair-color experience and has not yet been faced with having to overcome unwanted tones will have some difficulty understanding the effects of dimensional hair coloring.

SHUFFLING CARDS

Figure 27.1

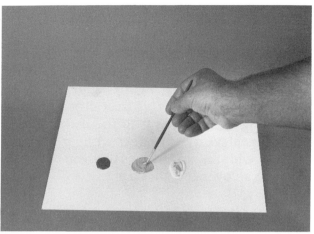

Place some light-colored and some dark-colored paint on a piece of white cardboard. Mix some of the light and dark color together to achieve a new color. Explain to your students that although many craftsmen and artisans who work with color have the ability to mix a lighter color with a darker color to achieve a variation in between, hair colorists do not have that luxury.

Figure 27.2

If we have a dark hair color, and we want to achieve a lighter color, it is often impossible to do because of undertones that are in the hair. You could end up with a hair color that is less than desirable because the tint does not have the ability to lighten the hair sufficiently. (Also refer to Chapter 22, "Categories of Natural Hair Color.")

By using bleach to lighten small segments of the hair you achieve a lighter effect by dispersing the light hair in with the darker hair. For the purpose of this experiment, the dark set of cards shown here indicates dark hair.

The light deck of cards represents the sections of hair that you would lighten with a bleach.

Figure 27.3

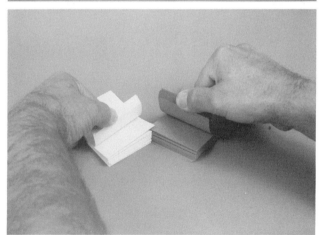

Shuffle the cards together as you would a deck of playing cards.

Figure 27.4

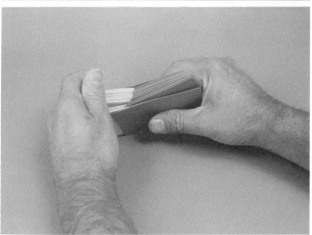

Shuffle the cards so that there are an equal number of light and dark cards in the deck.

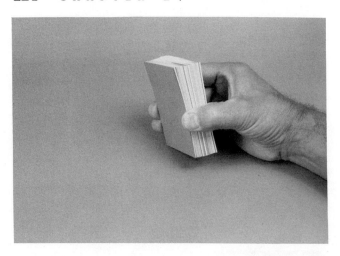

Figure 27.5

The cards are now mixed together. The purpose of this demonstration is to show your students that you can solve hair-color problems or achieve a slightly lighter or darker effect without having to treat all of the hair. By adding lighter strands to the darker strands you achieve a light effect without having to deal with the undertones that you would get with an overall color change.

CHAPTER 28
Dimensional Hair-Coloring Prop

It is important for students to know how to use foil for dimensional effects. It is important for your students to know that, by adding lighter or darker strands of hair, the overall hair color will have a lighter or darker appearance. Students should realize that having the ability to do dimensional hair coloring will catapult them to the top of their profession. Custom creative hair-coloring services are in great demand. Applying a single process hair color on your client's hair will not allow a hair colorist to achieve the most beautiful result. What you can attempt to do as a cosmetology instructor is help your students understand that professional hair coloring is not simply pouring hair color into an applicator bottle or bowl and applying it to the hair. Professional hair coloring is a creative, systematic way of applying color to the hair to preserve its condition and enhance its looks.

There are hundreds of variations in methods of applying foils to the hair. Each one will create its own effect. When applying foils for the purpose of doing dimensional hair coloring, I prefer to use the straight-line method or "slicing the hair," as many call it. I prefer this method for many reasons. First, it is the easiest to teach. I can say this with some authority. Having taught other methods, I feel that the straight-line method is the easiest to grasp. Second, you can keep the hair in better condition. You can also achieve a greater degree of lightness without having to lighten the hair as much. When making this statement I usually get some raised eyebrows. "How can you get the hair lighter without bleaching it more?" That is the primary reason for building the following prop. The prop will show, without a doubt, that you can achieve an overall lighter effect by taking thin slices of hair, as opposed to a thicker section, and weaving it.

The more you bunch the hair together when you lighten it, the darker the hair will appear. The more you spread this bunch of hair out among the natural hair, the lighter it will appear. It actually creates an optical illusion by the diffusion. When showing this prop the students will still have a difficult time understanding why the hair appears dark and light if it has been bleached to the same degree. You must be prepared to answer your skeptics. This is best accomplished by leaving one of the long strands intact, then folding it over to demonstrate how it darkens as it gets thicker.

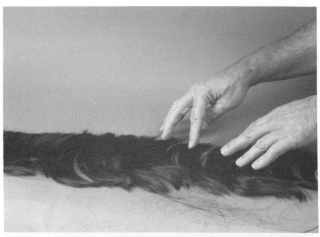

Figure 28.1

Spread out the hair that you are going to use. To make long strips of hair, spread the hair out to cover about 30 inches. For this prop, it is best if you use darker hair, because you want to show that it is possible to achieve a light look even with dark hair.

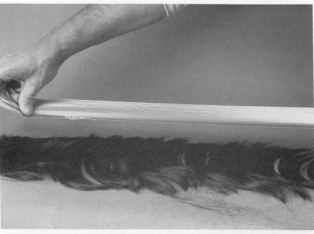

Figure 28.2

Pull off a piece of duct tape long enough to cover the entire length of the hair that is spread out.

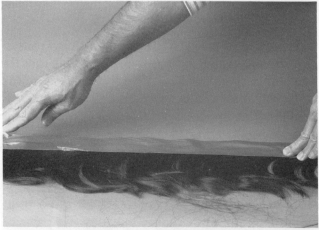

Figure 28.3

Place the tape down over the hair. Press firmly on the tape to make certain the hair has adhered to it.

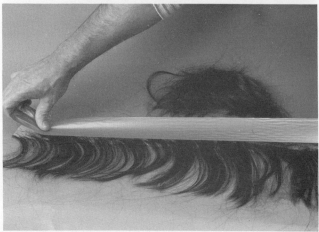

Figure 28.4

Flip the hair and the tape over and remove any excess hair that has not adhered to the tape. Set this hair aside; it can be used to make more long strands. Next place another piece of duct tape down, sandwiching the hair between two pieces of tape.

DIMENSIONAL HAIR-COLORING PROP   127

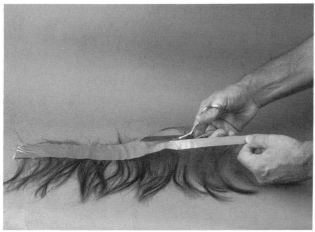

Figure 28.5

Cut the tape in half lengthwise, removing all of the excess, unnecessary tape.

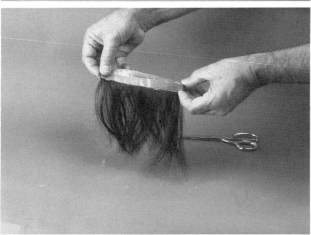

Figure 28.6

Fold the tape several times and line up the tape to make sure that the top of the tape is even.

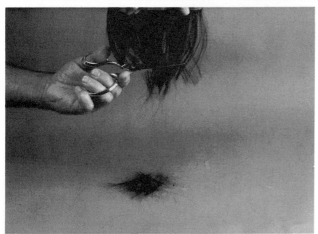

Figure 28.7

Cut the ends of the strands off so that they will be even.

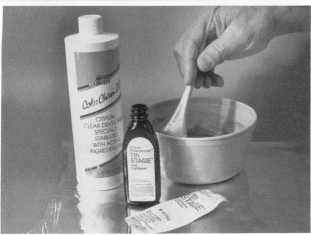

Figure 28.8

Mix a mild on-the-scalp bleach in a bowl. It is important that you bleach the hair slowly for a more uniform bleachout.

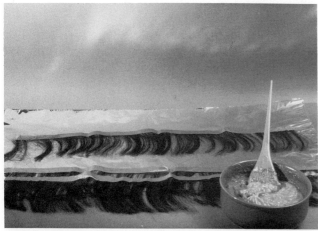

Figure 28.9
Place a large section of foil on a flat surface and then place the first strip of hair to be lightened on top of the foil.

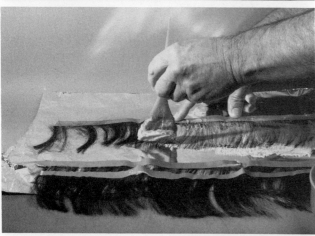

Figure 28.10
Apply the bleach on the hair generously. Flip the strand over and apply bleach to the other side.

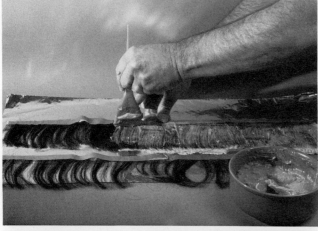

Figure 28.11
Place the second strip of hair directly over the first strand and repeat the process. Even though you are working with thin strips of hair, it is wise to flip the sections of hair over and reapply the bleach to make certain of uniform bleachout.

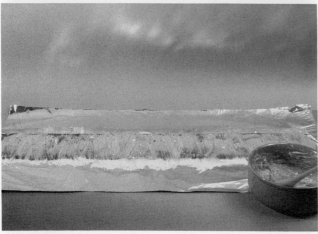

Figure 28.12
Allow the bleach to process for about 1 hour and 15 minutes. Shampoo the bleach off and reapply a freshly mixed bleach. The complete bleaching time for this dark hair will take at least 2 ½ hours. Do not attempt to speed the bleaching process up by using an excessively strong bleach. Remember, slower is better.

DIMENSIONAL HAIR-COLORING PROP 129

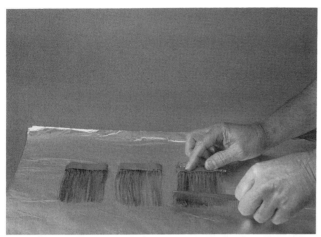

Figure 28.13
After the hair has lightened to a yellow stage, remove the bleach. Fold the strands over twice, comb out the tangles, and allow to dry.

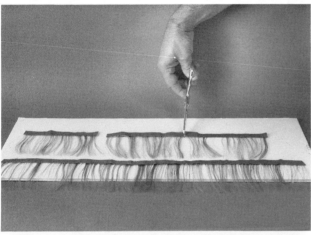

Figure 28.14
After the hair has dried, cut the long sections into six equal smaller sections.

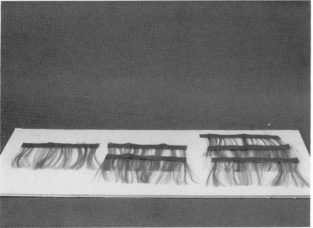

Figure 28.15
Lay the six sections out as shown. The first sections will be one strand thick, the second two strands thick, and the third three strands thick.

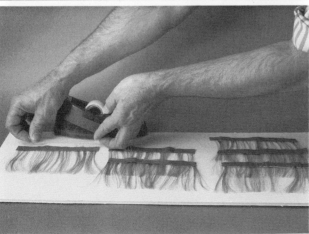

Figure 28.16
Using transparent tape, tape the sections down onto a piece of foam-core cardboard.

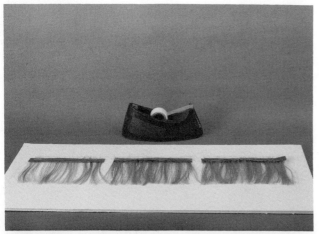

Figure 28.17
When the sections are taped down they should look like this.

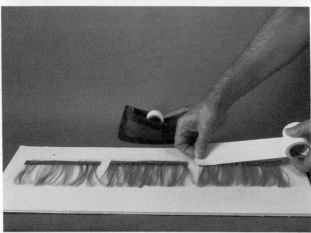

Figure 28.18
For a neater appearance place a piece of white cloth tape over the duct tape.

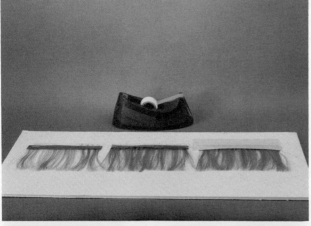

Figure 28.19
The white cloth tape covers the silver duct tape and gives the prop a more professional appearance.

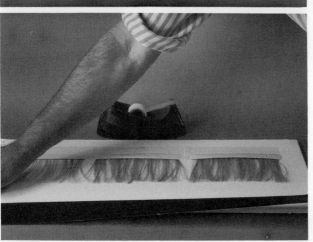

Figure 28.20
Border the prop with black cloth tape. This frames the prop and gives it more durability.

DIMENSIONAL HAIR-COLORING PROP 131

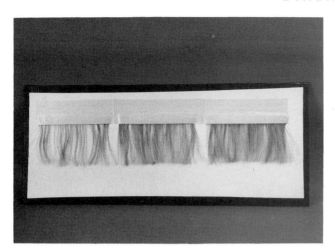

Figure 28.21
Here you have the finished prop. This prop will give your students a better understanding of why it is in their best interest to take thinner sections of hair if a lighter color is desired.

CHAPTER 29
Creating Different Hair Colors with Dimensional Hair Coloring

Dimensional hair color is the lifeblood of professional hair coloring. The better your students understand dimensional hair coloring, the greater their chances for success in the profession.

The following prop is designed to clearly show students the many facets of dimensional hair coloring and how this service can be used to change the ambiance of a client's hair color without making a total commitment.

Although we have only shown four different effects with this particular prop, the possibilities for variety are endless.

CREATING DIFFERENT HAIR COLORS WITH DIMENSIONAL HAIR COLORING 133

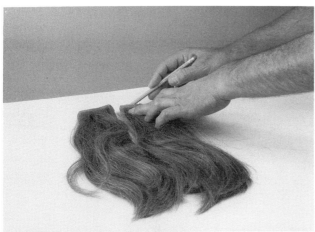

Figure 29.1

Determine how many sections of hair are to be used and lay them out on a foam-core board. For the prop, we are going to use sections of hair. You may elect to use mannequins to show the differences in color. It is important that all of the hair used be exactly the same color. Different hair colors will not give a true demonstration of how dimensional colors affect the hair.

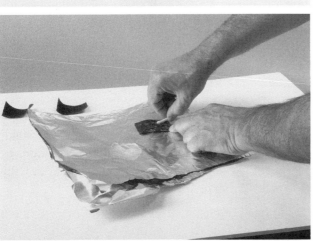

Figure 29.2

Once the layout is complete attach pieces of Velcro to the foam-core board, so that sections of hair can be removed from the board easily. It is important that you can remove the sections so that you can show the students the amount of hair that was treated to achieve the effect. Be certain to always leave one of the hair sections natural.

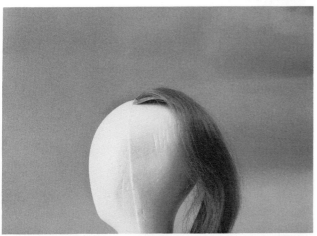

Figure 29.3

Determine how each of the sections are to be colored. Pin one of the sections to a foam head or a wig block. Be certain that the various coloring techniques that are to be used are different enough so that the differences can be clearly seen.

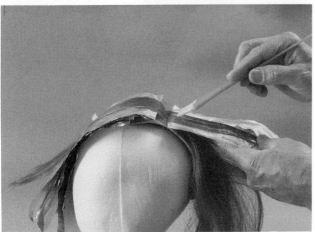

Figure 29.4

On this section of hair we are going to use bleach to lighten thin slices of hair. Apply bleach to the hair slices, the same as you would for the entire head.

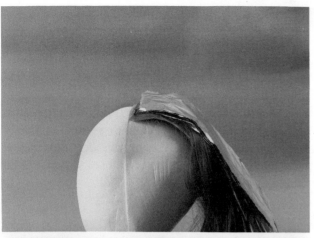

Figure 29.5
Continue working down the section until the desired number of foils have been applied. Allow to process until the hair has reached the stage of lightness desired. Shampoo, condition, and dry the hair. It is important that the treated sections feel and look as good as the section that is left untreated.

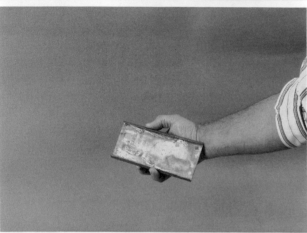

Figure 29.6
Because the Velcro will not adhere to the back of the sections and because it is necessary to remove and replace the sections from the foam-core board, we have prepared pieces of metal to hold the sections in place. These may be purchased from a sheet metal shop. Make certain that the shop that makes the pieces of metal for you deburrs the edges so that they are not sharp.

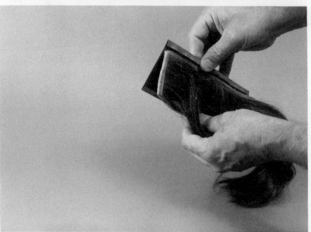

Figure 29.7
Fit the section of hair into the piece of metal. The edges of the metal should be pre-bent so that clamping the edges down over the section will be easy.

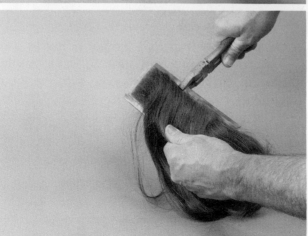

Figure 29.8
With a pair of pliers, clamp down the edges firmly over the section of hair. Once the section has been firmly clamped in place, adhere a piece of Velcro to the back of the metal to match the Velcro on the foam-core board.

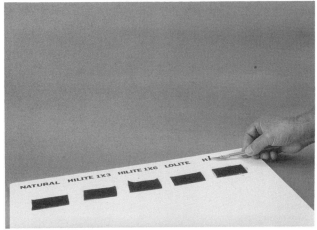

Figure 29.9

On the foam-core board, identify the dimensional hair-color techniques that were carried out on each section. On this particular prop, two of the sections were lightened, one was lightened in proportion of one section to three natural sections, another was lightened in proportion of one section to six natural sections, another was low-lightened, and yet another was high-low lightened.

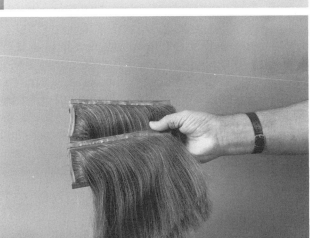

Figure 29.10

Remove the section from the board and hold it on the side so that you can clearly see the ratio of colored hair to natural hair. In this way, the student will be able to better anticipate the changes that can be accomplished by the use of dimensional hair coloring.

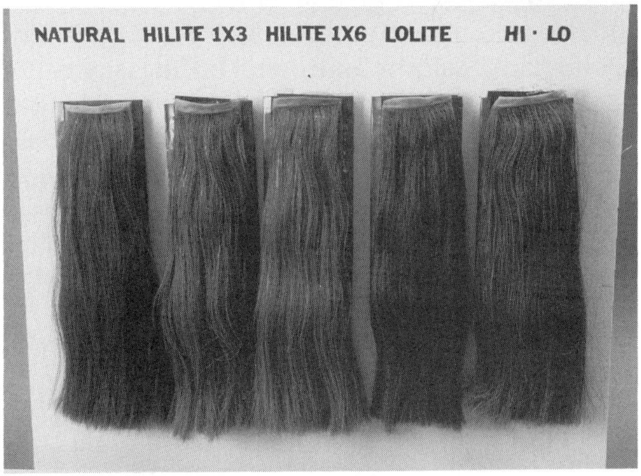

Fig. 29.11

The finished prop can be mounted on the wall or stored safely until it is time to present a lecture on "the advantages of dimensional hair coloring."

CHAPTER 30

Coloring Gray Hair

No one has really ever determined why hair turns gray. Stories have circulated as long as there has been gray hair. "Her hair turned gray overnight when she was frightened by a near accident," someone will say. Or "One morning she woke up and her hair was all gray, and for no reason." These kinds of stories have been passed on for years. No one really knows why hair turns gray when it does, although there is strong evidence that it is primarily genetic. That is to say, if the parents' hair showed early signs of graying, chances are that the children's hair will also age prematurely. Some would argue that attitudes are changing, but gray hair is still associated with aging and dullness.

Individuals in today's society are constantly being bombarded by media ads for methods to remain youthful looking. People seek ways to look younger. Politicians, salespeople, and businessmen and -women are all under pressure to look more youthful. Many do their own hair color at home with a fair degree of success, but home hair coloring is limited. Special effects and advanced techniques cannot be achieved by an untrained person. This is why home hair color will never replace professional hair coloring.

Gray hair can be a curse, or it can be a blessing. When it comes to hair color, it is certainly most often the catalyst that pushes the client to color his or her hair. For the hair colorist that is a blessing. On the other hand it can also complicate the hair-color service. Gray hair will not respond to hair coloring the same way as the natural color hair, but they will both be on the same head. This is why gray hair offers challenges to the hair colorist that would not otherwise exist.

What occurs during the graying process? The melanin in the hair shaft loses color. The melanin is still there, nestled in the cortex of the hair shaft, the same as it would be if there was color in it; it is just colorless. If you bleach the hair that is void of color the melanin is still disrupted. It still dissolves the same as a colored segment of melanin. The strand would become weakened, the cuticle would be lifted, and the hair would become more porous. The hair color could also take on a yellow cast. This same yellow cast can also result from other causes, such as smoking, medication, exposure to the sun, and, to a lesser degree, hair sprays and styling aids.

There are at least as many varieties of gray hair as there are colors of hair. Presently there is no well-defined method of identifying gray hair. First the amount of gray hair is determined (the actual percentage of gray hairs on the head). Second, determine the location of those gray hairs (where the gray hairs are located on the head). One person who is 50 percent gray could have the gray hair sprinkled equally throughout the hair; another could have the same amount of gray hair located in the front portion of the head. Each of these factors would require a different approach to hair-color formulating.

Another consideration when formulating a hair color to cover gray hair is the color of the client's hair before it turned gray. The hair colorist must recognize that when the hair starts to turn gray the remaining natural hair changes as well. It is difficult for even the accomplished hair colorist to identify the level of the client's natural hair once the hair has turned substantially gray. Gray hair does a masterful job of concealing the undertones that remain in the hair. The undertones are still there, and they are no less intense than they were before the hair turned gray. This is why we introduce the system of identifying the natural hair colors by using the category system.

Let us explore what each natural hair-color category goes through when the hair starts to turn gray. Individuals in the B category, dark brown and black, go through the least change when the hair begins to turn gray. The hair is generally on the cool side, so there is no major change in the natural hair color when the hair grays. Clients in this category offer the greatest challenge to the hair colorist. The hair colorist must determine when you no longer color the gray hair dark to match the natural hair color. At some point in the client's life she or he can no longer continue to wear the dark hair colors as when he or she was younger. At this point the hair colorist must lighten the hair and at the same time minimize the red/orange tones that are generally unflattering to the client in this category. The red tones that this client can wear most successfully are the blue/red tones.

In the W category, warm brown, the hair goes through dramatic changes as the hair begins to turn gray. Even before the hair begins to gray the natural hair color loses its warmth and starts to flatten. As more and more gray hair appears the natural color continues to lose its warmth until it becomes an ashy tone. What the hair colorist must remember is that the undertones that were there before the hair turned gray are still there. Clients in this category offer the hair colorist a challenge, but not as great a challenge as clients in the B category. This category of client grew up with warm hair. He or she is more accustomed to seeing red tones in the hair, and therefore when the hair color is returned to a warm tone it is not as traumatic to the client. This client can generally wear red tones very well and often requests it. This client also wears highlights very well. When you ask clients about how their hair color responded to the sun during summer vacations in high school they will reveal some facts about how their hair lightened. They will say, "My hair turned an attractive golden tone when I went out into the sun." Or they may say, "I didn't like the color of my hair when I went out into the sun;

it turned an awful red tone." Remember, when you consult with clients listen very carefully to their replies to your questions. Some clients do not realize how much their hair color has changed since it started turning gray, so you should say that you want to return their hair to the same glow it had when they were in high school.

The S category, soft brown, is the category whose hair grays the least gracefully. The natural hair is light and does not make an attractive contrast when the hair color begins to gray. The color usually takes on a drab, dreary look. This category is generally not as challenging because it does not have the red/orange undertones that the B and W categories contain. This category of hair color is the only one that a single-process blonde can be used on. You should not hesitate to make this client blonde when he or she begins to turn gray. Remember, people in this category were usually blonde during high school, so they are generally not averse to once again becoming a blonde. Care must be taken when you lighten this client's hair for the first time. Remember that the hair lightens faster at the scalp. When you use a high-lift tint you will get an unnatural look if the ends are darker than the scalp. It is more practical to lift the color from the hair by bleaching the hair for the first time, then maintaining the hair color with a high-lift tint.

The R category, red, like the S category, does not gray gracefully. The once vibrant red hair starts to lose its color when the hair begins to turn gray. It becomes a muddy red color. It is usually easy to convince people in this category that they should cover their gray hair and restore the vibrancy to the hair. It is hard to believe, but many times changes in hair color happen so gradually that the client may not realize that once vibrant red hair is losing its glow. This client does not offer a great challenge. They generally just want their hair restored to its original tone.

You can see the importance of knowing what a client's hair color was as a child and during young adult years. Knowing this will give you a strong indication of the hair-color formula that is best suited for your client. Mother nature is never wrong! Once you establish the natural hair-color category it will also help to better evaluate the skin tone.

FORMULATING FOR GRAY HAIR

The gray card shown in Figure 30.1 is used in the television industry, photo industry, and in graphic arts to measure increments of gray from black to pure white. For our purposes the numbering has been changed so that it conforms to the level system in the hair-coloring industry. This gray card will help you to develop formulas for coloring hair that is turning gray. The basic rule for formulating for gray hair is as follows. If you have 30 percent gray hair and 70 percent natural the total for these is 100 percent. Easy so far. We will assume that the gray hair is distributed throughout the hair evenly. You will use the gray card now to help you formulate. The gray hair will be considered white on the gray card. The natural hair will be determined on the gray chart by the category of natural hair color; for instance someone in the B category will be a level one. Someone in the W category will be considered level two. The S category will be considered level three on the gray card. The reason that we give different levels to the different categories is that the natural color is a darker color. Let us assume now that the client has 30 percent gray hair and 70 percent natural and is in the warm brown category (Figs. 30.2 and 30.3). That would make her natural hair color a number two on the gray chart. Now you would add three parts to her natural level (two) plus three, which is 30 percent gray, and you end up with a number five on the gray card. This is the natural level of hair color that you should attempt to achieve.

The level on the gray card is the level that you want to reach, not the level of hair color that you want to use. This system of formulating for gray hair is used to figure out the percentage of gray that the client is used to seeing. This gray hair gives the client the perception of having lighter hair. This method of formulating is a method of determining how much lighter you should make the client's hair to give the illusion of lightness that he or she is accustomed to.

Take another example of someone in the B category (Figs. 30.4 and 30.5). This client has a sprinkling of gray hair (less than 5 percent). You can see that, in this case, you could feel safe in coloring the hair back to its natural hair color. The client would have to have at least 10 percent gray before it is necessary to lighten the natural level. This is determined by the amount of gray hair the client is accustomed to seeing. Even though she has a small gray streak in the front of her hair you can feel safe in coloring her hair close to her natural hair color.

Let us look at one more example. This client is in the soft brown category (Figs. 30.6 and 30.7). He has 20 percent gray hair. You start with a level three (soft brown is level three), add 2 (the percentage of gray hair), and you end up with a level five. You would make this client's hair a level five. If the client had 30 percent gray hair, you would add yet another number, leaving you with a level six.

When you are determing formulas, look at your client as though her hair color was a black-and-white photograph. Then try to achieve the same level with hair coloring (Figs. 30.8 and 30.9).

When you are faced with a situation where the amount of gray dictates that you should lighten the hair to reach a certain level of color, and yet you know that if you attempted to lighten the hair to that degree you would get some undesirable undertones in the remaining natural hair, you must be creative in your color mixing. For example, you could use a darker hair color that will not lighten the hair to bring out the undesirable undertones, then achieve lightness by adding some highlights to the hair. A variety of techniques can help solve your hair-color challenges. The more problem-solving techniques you have at your disposal, the greater latitude you will have. Remember, your knowledge and techniques are your tools for successful hair coloring.

Study each of the clients shown in this chapter and note what formulation and technique was used to achieve the end color result. This will help you establish some guidelines for yourself. Learning hair color is not a destination; it is a journey that never ends.

CHAPTER 30

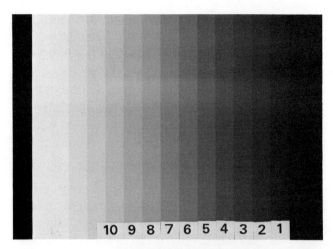

Figure 30.1
The gray card.

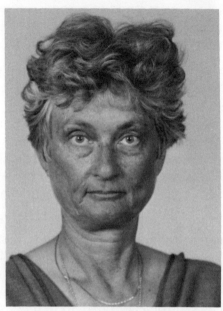

Figure 30.2
A client in the S category (warm brown category) with 30 percent gray hair and 70 percent natural.

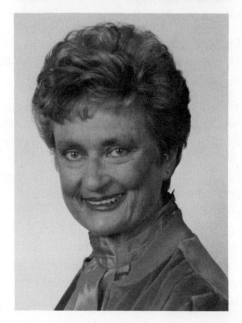

Figure 30.3
The same client after hair-color formulation.

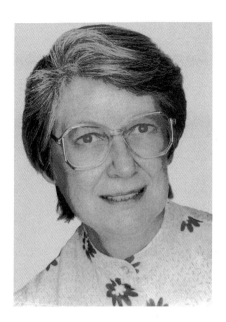

Figure 30.4

A client in the B category with a sprinkling of gray hair (less than 5 percent).

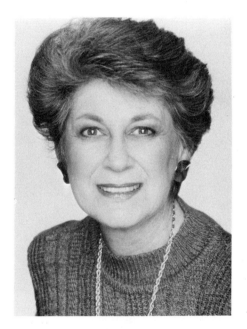

Figure 30.5

The same client after hair-color formulation.

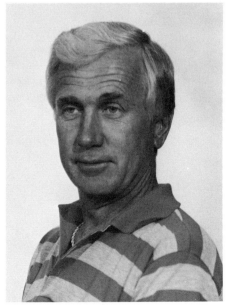

Figure 30.6

A client in the soft brown category with 20 percent gray hair.

142 CHAPTER 30

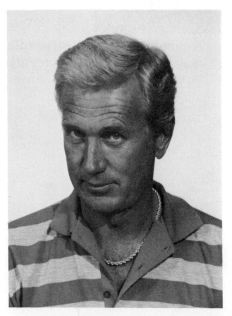

Figure 30.7
The same client after hair-color formulation.

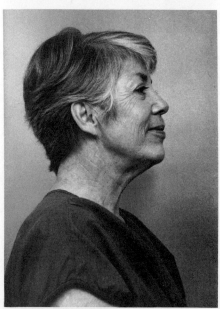

Figure 30.8
A client before hair-color formulation.

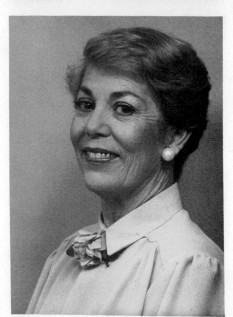

Figure 30.9
The same client after hair-color formulation.

COLORING GRAY HAIR

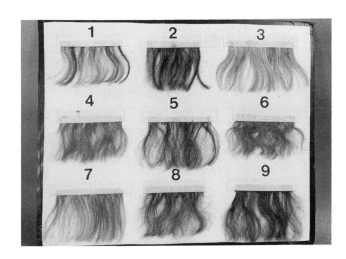

Figure 30.10

When you look at and study the gray hair shown on this chart you will note that there are as many types and distributions of gray hair as there are natural hair colors. Each one presents a special challenge. Handle each first-time client with consideration. This is a difficult decision.

Hair Coloring Glossary

accelerator: (See *activator*.)

accent color: A concentrated color product that can be added to permanent, semi-permanent, or temporary hair color to intensify or tone down the color. Another word for *concentrate*.

acid: An aqueous (water-based) solution with a pH less than 7.0 on the pH scale.

activator: An additive used to quicken the action or progress of a chemical. Another word for *booster, accelerator, protenator,* or *catalyst*.

alkaline: An aqueous (water-based) solution with a pH greater than 7.0 on the pH scale. The opposite of acid.

allergy: A reaction due to extreme sensitivity to certain foods or chemicals.

allergy test: A test to determine the possibility or degree of sensitivity, also known as a patch test, predisposition test, or skin test.

amino acids: The group of molecules that the body uses to synthesize protein. There are 22 different amino acids found in living protein that serve as units of structure in protein.

ammonia: A colorless pungent gas composed of hydrogen and nitrogen; in water solution it is called ammonia water. Used in hair color to swell the cuticle. When mixed with hydrogen peroxide, activates the oxidation process on melanin and allows the melanin to decolorize.

ammonium hydroxide: An alkali solution of ammonia in water, commonly used in the manufacture of permanent hair color, lightener preparations, and hair relaxers.

analysis (hair): An examination of the hair to determine its condition and natural color. (See *consultation; condition.*)

aqueous: Descriptive term for water solution or any medium that is largely composed of water.

ash: A tone or shade dominated by greens, blues, violets, or grays. May be used to counteract unwanted warm tones.

base (alkali): (See *pH; alkaline.*)

base color: (See *color base.*)

bleeding: Seepage of tint/lightener from foil or cap due to improper application.

HAIR COLORING GLOSSARY 145

blending:	A merging of one tint or tone with another.
blonding:	A term applied to the lightening of the hair.
bonds:	The means by which atoms are joined together to make molecules.
booster:	(See *activator.*)
brassy tone:	Red, orange, or gold tones in the hair.
breakage:	A condition in which hair splits and breaks off.
build-up:	Repeated coatings on the hair shaft.
catalyst:	A substance used to alter the speed of a chemical reaction.
caustic:	Strongly alkaline materials. At very high pH levels, can burn or destroy protein or tissue by chemical action.
certified color:	A color that meets certain standards for purity and is certified by the FDA.
cetyl alcohol:	Fatty alcohol used as an emollient. It is also used as a stabilizer for emulsion systems and in hair color and cream developer as a thickener.
chelating stabilizer:	A molecule that binds metal ions and renders them inactive.
chemical change:	Alteration in the chemical composition of a substance.
citric acid:	Organic acid derived from citrus fruits and used for pH adjustment. Primarily used to adjust the acid-alkali balance. Has some antioxidant and preservative qualities. Used medicinally as a mild astringent.
coating:	Residue left on the outside of the hair shaft.
color:	Visual sensation caused by light.
color additive:	(See *accent color.*)
color base:	The combination of dyes that make up the tonal foundation of a specific hair color.
color mixing:	Combining two or more shades for a custom color.
color refresher:	1. Color applied to midshaft and ends to give a more uniform color appearance to the hair. 2. Color applied by a shampoo-in method to enhance the natural color. Also called color wash, color enhancer.
color remover:	A product designed to remove artificial pigment from the hair.
color test:	The process of removing product from a hair strand to monitor the progress of color development during tinting for lightening.
color wheel:	The arrangement of primary, secondary, and tertiary colors in the order of their relationships to each other. A tool for formulating.
complementary colors:	Primary and secondary colors positioned opposite each other on the color wheel. When these two colors are combined, they create a neutral color. Combinations are as follows: blue/orange, red/green, yellow/violet.
concentrate:	(See *accent color.*)
condition:	The existing state of the hair; elasticity, strength, texture, porosity, and evidence of previous treatments.
consultation:	Verbal communication with a client to determine desired result. (See *analysis, hair.*)

contributing pigment:	The current level and tone of the hair; refers to both natural contributing pigment and decolorized (or lightened) contributing pigment. (See *undertone.*)
cool tones:	(See *ash.*)
corrective coloring:	The process of correcting an undesirable color.
cortex:	The second layer of hair. A fibrous protein core of the hair fiber, containing melanin pigment.
coverage:	Reference to the ability of a color product to color gray, white, or other colors of hair.
cuticle:	The translucent protein outer layer of the hair fiber.
cysteic acid:	A chemical substance in the hair fiber, produced by the interaction of hydrogen peroxide on the disulfide bond (cysteine).
cysteine:	The disulfide amino acid that joins protein chains together.
D & C colors:	Colors selected from a certified list approved by the Food and Drug Administration for use in drug and cosmetic products.
decolorize:	A chemical process involving the lightening of the natural color pigment or artificial color from the hair.
degree:	Term used to describe various units of measurement.
dense:	Thick, compact, or crowded.
deposit:	Describes a color product in terms of its ability to add color pigment to the hair. Color added equals deposit.
deposit only color:	A category of color products between permanent and semipermanent colors. Formulated to deposit color, not lift. They contain oxidation dyes and utilize low volume developer.
depth:	The lightness or darkness of a specific hair color. (See *value; level.*)
developer:	An oxidizing agent, usually hydrogen peroxide, that reacts chemically with coloring material to develop color molecules and create a change in natural hair color.
development time (oxidation period):	The time required for a permanent color or lightener to completely develop.
diffused:	Broken down, scattered; not limited to one spot.
direct dye:	A pre-formed color that dyes the fiber directly without the need for oxidation.
discoloration:	The development of undesired shades through chemical reaction.
double process:	A technique requiring two separate procedures in which the hair is decolorized or pre-lightened with a lightener before the depositing color is applied.
drab:	Term used to describe hair color shades containing no red or gold. (See *ash; dull.*)
drabber:	Concentrated color, used to reduce red or gold highlights.
dull:	A word used to describe hair or hair color without sheen.
dye:	Artificial pigment.
dye intermediate:	A material that develops into color only after reaction with developer (hydrogen peroxide). Also known as oxidation dyes.

dye solvents or dye remover:	(See *color remover*.)
dye stock:	(See *color base*.)
elasticity:	The ability of the hair to stretch and return to normal.
enzyme:	A protein molecule found in living cells that initiates a chemical process.
fade:	To lose color through exposure to the elements or other factors.
fillers:	1. Color product used as a color refresher or to fill damaged hair in preparation for hair coloring. 2. Any liquid-like substance to help fill a void. (See *color refresher*.)
formulas:	Mixtures of two or more ingredients.
formulate:	The art of mixing to create a blend or balance of two or more ingredients.
gray hair:	Hair with decreasing amounts of natural pigment. Hair with no natural pigment is actually white. White hair looks gray when mingled with the still-pigmented hair.
hair:	A slender, thread-like outgrowth of the skin of the head and body.
hair root:	That part of the hair contained within the follicle, below the surface of the scalp.
hair shaft:	Visible part of each strand of hair. It is made up of an outer layer called the cuticle, an innermost layer called the medulla, and an in-between layer called the cortex. The cortex layer is where color changes are made.
hard water:	Water that contains minerals and metallic salts as impurities.
henna:	A plant-extracted coloring that produces bright shades of red. The active ingredient is lawsone. Henna permanently colors the hair by coating and penetrating the hair shaft. (See *progressive dye*.)
high lift tinting:	A single-process color treatment with a higher degree of lightening action and a minimal amount of color deposit.
highlighting:	The introduction of a lighter color in small, selected sections to increase hair lightness. Generally not strongly contrasting from the natural color.
hydrogen peroxide:	An oxidizing chemical made up of 2 parts hydrogen and 2 parts oxygen (H_2O_2), used to aid the processing of permanent hair color and lighteners. Also referred to as a developer; available in liquid or cream.
level:	A unit of measurement, used to evaluate the lightness or darkness of a color, excluding tone.
level system:	In hair coloring, a system colorists use to analyze the lightness or darkness of a hair color.
lift:	The lightening actions of a hair color or lightening products on the hair's natural pigment.
lightener:	The chemical compound that lightens the hair by dispersing, dissolving, and decolorizing the natural hair pigment. (See *pre-lighten*.)
lightening:	(See *decolorize*.)

line of demarcation:	An obvious difference between two colors on the hair shaft.
litmus paper:	A chemically treated paper used to test the acidity or alkalinity of products.
medulla:	The center structure of the hair shaft. Very little is known about its actual function.
melanin:	The tiny grains of pigment in the hair cortex that create natural hair color.
melanocytes:	Cells in the hair bulb that manufacture melanin.
melanoprotein:	The protein coating of a melanosome.
melanosome:	Protein-coated granule containing melanin.
metallic dyes:	Soluble metal salts, such as lead, silver, and bismuth, which produce colors on the hair fiber by progressive build-up and exposure to air.
modifier:	A chemical found as an ingredient in permanent hair colors. Its function is to alter the dye intermediates.
molecule:	Two or more atoms chemically joined together; the smallest part of a compound.
neutral:	1. A color balanced between warm and cool, which does not reflect a highlight of any primary or secondary color. 2. Also refers to a pH of 7.
neutralization:	The process that counterbalances or cancels the action of an agent or color.
neutralize:	Render neutral; counterbalance of action or influence. (See *neutral*.)
new growth:	The part of the hair shaft that is between previously chemically treated hair and the scalp.
nonalkaline:	(See *acid*.)
off-the-scalp lightener:	Generally a stronger lightener, usually in powder form, not to be used directly on the scalp.
on-the-scalp lightener:	A liquid, cream, or gel form of lightener that can be used directly on the scalp.
opaque:	Allowing no light to shine through.
outgrowth:	(See *new growth*.)
overlap:	Occurs when the application of color or lightener goes beyond the line of demarcation.
over-porosity:	The condition when hair reaches an undesirable stage of porosity, requiring correction.
oxidation:	1. The reaction of dye intermediates with hydrogen peroxide found in hair-coloring developers. 2. The interaction of hydrogen peroxide on the natural pigment.
oxidative hair color:	A product containing oxidation dyes, which requires hydrogen peroxide to develop the permanent color.
para tint:	A tint made from oxidation dyes.
para-phenylenediamine:	An oxidation dye used in most permanent hair colors, often abbreviated as P.P.D.

patch test:	A test required by the Food and Drug Act. Made by applying a small amount of the hair coloring preparation to the skin of the arm or behind the ear to determine possible allergies (hypersensitivity). Also called predisposition or skin test.
penetrating color:	Color that enters or penetrates the cortex or second layer of the hair shaft.
permanent color:	1. Hair-color products that do not wash out by shampooing. 2. A category of hair-color products mixed with developer that create a lasting color change.
peroxide:	(See *hydrogen peroxide*.)
peroxide residue:	Traces of peroxide left in the hair after treatment with lightener or tint.
persulfate:	In hair coloring, a chemical ingredient commonly used in activators. It increases the speed of the decolorization process. (See *activator*.)
pH:	The quantity that expresses the acid/alkali balance. A pH of 7 is the neutral value for pure water. Any pH below 7 is acidic; any pH above 7 is alkaline. The skin is mildly acidic and generally in the pH 4.5 to 5.5 range.
pH scale:	A numerical scale from 0 (very acid) to 14 (very alkaline), used to describe the degree of acidity or alkalinity.
pigment:	Any substance or matter used as coloring: natural or artificial hair color.
porosity:	Ability of the hair to absorb water or other liquids.
powder lightener:	(See *off the scalp lightener*.)
pre-bleaching:	(See *pre-lighten*.)
predisposition test:	(See *patch test*.)
pre-lighten:	Generally the first step of double-process hair coloring, used to lift or lighten the natural pigment. (See *decolorize*.)
pre-soften:	The process of treating gray or very resistant hair to allow for better penetration of color.
primary colors:	Pigments or colors that are fundamental and cannot be made by mixing colors together. Red, yellow, and blue are the primary colors.
prism:	A transparent glass or crystal solid that breaks up white light into its component colors, the spectrum.
processing time:	The time required for the chemical treatment to react on the hair.
progressive dyes or progressive dye system:	1. A coloring system that produces increased absorption with each application. 2. Color products that deepen or increase absorption over a period of time during processing.
regrowth:	(See *new growth*.)
resistant hair:	Hair that is difficult to penetrate with moisture or chemical solutions.
retouch:	Application of color or lightening mixture to new growth of hair.
salt and pepper:	The descriptive term for a mixture of dark and gray or white hair.

secondary color:	Colors made by combining two primary colors in equal proportion; green, orange, and violet are secondary colors.
semi-permanent hair coloring:	Hair coloring that lasts through several shampoos. It penetrates the hair shaft and stains the cuticle layer, slowly diffusing out with each shampoo.
sensitivity:	A skin highly reactive to the presence of a specific chemical. Skin reddens or becomes irritated shortly after application of the chemical. On removal of the chemical, the reaction subsides.
shade:	1. A term used to describe a specific color. 2. The visible difference between two colors.
sheen:	The ability of the hair to shine, gleam, or reflect light.
single-process color:	Refers to an oxidative tint solution that lifts or lightens while also depositing color in one application. (See *oxidative hair color.*)
softening agent:	A mild alkaline product applied prior to the color treatment, to increase porosity, swell the cuticle layer of the hair, and increase color absorption. Tint that has not been mixed with developer is frequently used. (See *pre-soften.*)
solution:	A blended mixture of solid, liquid, or gaseous substances in a liquid medium.
solvent:	Carrier liquid in which other components may be dissolved.
specialist:	One who concentrates on one part or branch of a subject or profession.
spectrum:	The series of colored bands diffracted and arranged in the order of their wavelengths by the passage of white light through a prism. Shading continuously from red (produced by the longest wave visible) to violet (produced by the shortest): red, orange, yellow, blue, indigo, and violet.
spot lightening:	Color correcting using a lightening mixture to lighten darker areas.
stabilizer:	General name for ingredient that prolongs lifetime, appearance, and performance of a product.
stage:	A term used to describe a visible color change that natural hair color goes through while being lightened.
stain remover:	Chemical used to remove tint stains from skin.
strand test:	Test given before treatment to determine development time, color result, and the ability of the hair to withstand the effects of chemicals.
stripping:	(See *color remover.*)
surfactant:	A short way of saying surface active agent. A molecule that is composed of an oil-loving (oleophilic) part and a water-loving (hydrophilic) part. They act as a bridge to allow oil and water to mix. Wetting agents, emulsifiers, cleansers, solubilizers, dispersing aids, and thickeners are usually surfactants.
tablespoon:	1/2 of an ounce. 3 teaspoons. 15 milliliters.
teaspoon:	1/6 of an ounce. 1/3 of a tablespoon. 5 milliliters.

temporary coloring or temporary rinses:	Color made from pre-formed dyes that are applied to the hair, but are readily removed with shampoo.
terminology:	The special words or terms used in science, art, or business.
tertiary colors:	The mixture of a primary and an adjacent secondary color on the color wheel. Red-orange, yellow-orange, yellow-green, blue-green, blue-violet, red-violet. Also referred to as intermediary colors.
texture, hair:	The diameter of an individual hair strand. Termed: coarse, medium, or fine.
tint:	Permanent oxidizing hair color product with the ability to lift and deposit color in the same process.
tint back:	To return hair to its original or natural color.
tone:	A term used to describe warmth or coolness in color.
toner:	A pastel color to be used after pre-lightening.
toning:	Adding color to modify the end result.
touch-up:	(See *retouch*.)
translucent:	The property of letting diffused light pass through.
tyrosinase:	The enzyme (tyrosinase) that reacts with the amino acid (tyrosine) to form the hair's natural melanin.
tyrosine:	The amino acid (tyrosine) that reacts with the enzyme (tyrosinase) to form the hair's natural melanin.
undertone:	The underlying color that emerges during the lifting process of melanin, which contributes to the end result. When lightening the hair, a residual warmth in tone always occurs.
urea peroxide:	A peroxide compound occasionally used in hair color. When added to an alkaline color mixture, it releases oxygen.
value:	(See *level; depth*.)
vegetable color:	A color derived from plant sources.
virgin hair:	Natural hair that has not undergone any chemical or physical abuse.
viscosity:	A term referring to the thickness of the solution.
volume:	The concentration of hydrogen peroxide in water solution. Expressed as volumes of oxygen liberated per volume of solution. 20 volume peroxide would thus liberate 20 pints (9.4 liters) of oxygen gas for each pint (liter) of solution.
warm:	Containing red, orange, yellow, or gold tones.